Mi Dor Le Dor

Genetics and Genetic Diseases: Jewish Legal and Ethical Perspectives

Mi Dor Le Dor

Genetics and Genetic Diseases: Jewish Legal and Ethical Perspectives

Deena R. Zimmerman, MD, MPH

KTAV Publishing House, Inc.

OUPRESS

KTAV Publishing House, Inc.
888 Newark Avenue
Jersey City, NJ 07306
Tel. (201) 963-9524
Fax. (201) 963-0102
www.ktav.com
bernie@ktav.com

OU Press
an imprint of the Orthodox Union
11 Broadway
New York, NY 10004
www.oupress.org
oupress@ou.org

Dedication

This book is dedicated to the memory of Yair Leibowitz
(Shevat 4, 5744–Tevet 14, 5761)
who taught me what it means to LIVE with a genetic disease.

Table of Contents

Section III: Living with Genetic Diseases

Acknowledgements

Many writers have used the analogy of writing to help describe the DNA code—each nucleotide is a letter, a codon is a word, and a strand of DNA is a sentence. I would like to use the reverse analogy—writing a book is similar to the biological process that is needed to pass information down from generation to generation. Like conception, it is not something that can be done alone; like replication, it starts with a backbone provided by the previous generation; and as with mutation, mistakes can creep in along the way.

The credit for the conception of this book goes to Bernie Scharfstein of Ktav Publishing House. He was the one with the insight to see that no book integrating medical and halachic aspects of genetics had yet been written, and that it was important that such a book be written. Mr. Scharfstein approached Rabbanit Chana Henkin, the Dean of Nishmat, The Jeanie Schottenstein Center for Advanced Torah Study for Women, and she approached me. Over the year-plus of writing the book, it became clear to me that he was correct. I want to thank him for the tremendous learning opportunity I had while writing this book, and thank Rabbanit Henkin for passing down to me the Jewish learning skills needed for the more halachic aspects of this book.

The process of writing the book was similar to a pregnancy. Those who know me personally know that this means it was not easy. Genetics is an enormous topic and one that has expanded exponentially over the last decade. Most of what I wrote in this book was unknown at the time I graduated medical school in 1988. However, Hashem does not create an illness before he creates the cure.[1] In this same time interval, the tools for doing research have expanded dramatically. For the first paper I wrote, I did research by searching shelves full of the *index medicus* in a medical school library.[2] At the time this book was written, research could be done in locations as diverse as Camp Morasha in Lake Como, Pennsylvania (while I was working as a camp doctor), and TEREM Emergency Medical Centers in Modiin, Israel, by my searching PubMed and Google via wireless internet. Because not all full articles are available without subscription, my thanks go to my TEREM research assistant, Dr. Baruch Hain, for providing me with the hundreds of full text articles (via the email that was not widely used in 1988) that were read in researching this volume.

To continue the analogy, childbirth is safer when attended by a skilled practitioner. The midwife of this project was Ilana Sober Elzufon, a fellow *yoetzet halacha* (and Yale graduate) who is also an amazing editor. Not only did she perform DNA repair on the multiple mutations I created in the English language, she provided many important insights that were incorporated into this book. They are too numerous to list individually, but she deserves credit for much content as well as style. Thanks are due to the editors of Ktav Publishing House as well.

My thanks to those authors who contributed chapters—Drs. Yoav Merrick, Isack Kandel, Alan Jotkowitz, Nicole Schreiber-Agus. and Matthew Cohen—for taking time from their very busy schedules to make the contributions.

I want to thank all those people whom I interviewed in writing the section on raising special children. They include both parents of special children and professionals who treat them. Most asked to remain anonymous. I will honor their requests but will emphasize how important their help was. I will particularly mention Chaye Lamm Warburg, who sat with me for a long time sharing her experience as the Director of Pediatric Occupational Therapy Services in Teaneck, New Jersey. I want also to thank all those who agreed to read parts of this book and share their insights. Particular thanks to Dr. Stephen Reingold, fellow pediatrician, who actually read the entire document. Special thanks to Rabbi Yehuda Henkin and Rabbi Reuven Aberman for reading the halachic sections of this work. Any remaining mistakes are my own.

Writing this book was a "generation to generation" experience for me. I had the pleasure of receiving assistance in the writing of a few chapters from some of my former students. Both Penina Dienstag and Melissa Meyers were students in the behavioral science small group that I led for a number of years for the New York Program of the Tel Aviv University Sackler School of Medicine. Penina is also a fellow *yoetzet halacha*. Penina played a crucial role in getting the project started, and Melissa helped in keeping it going.

Going to the *pshat*[3] of this analogy, I want to thank my partner in producing my real next generation, my husband Rabbi Sammy Zimmerman. He has put up with all my birth pains both literally and figuratively. My children, Ari, Akiva, Rivka, Yosef, and Tikva, deserve thanks for all the time they put up with being ignored because "Ima is working on her book." My daughter material used for the book, and Ari for always asking how I was coming along. I thank the previous generation, my parents and in-laws, as well.

Last, and certainly not least, my thanks to Hashem for giving me the strength to complete endeavors such as this, as well as functioning from day to day.

---

1. Talmud Bavli Megillah 13b
2. For the younger generation out there, this was an annual list of periodical articles.
3. The "simple meaning" of the text, or in this case the analogy.

Introduction:
Why a Book on Genetics and Judaism?

Genetics is a science that affects us all. Our genes are responsible for our basic physical makeup and ongoing function. When something goes wrong, then we are left with "genetic diseases." A number of these conditions are associated with a Jewish family background and thus are sometimes known as "Jewish genetic diseases."

Furthermore, genetics is a growing science that continues to raise many ethical challenges. It is important to understand what Jewish tradition can contribute to the debates regarding these challenges—both for those who follow Jewish law (*halacha*) and for those who wish to examine the Jewish perspective as a potential paradigm for general medical ethics.

The goal of the book is thus multifaceted:

1. To provide an up-to-date overview of the science of human genetics and its impact on human health. We acknowledge at the outset that producing a completely up-to-date work is impossible; the pace of growth of this science is faster than the process of publication. Nevertheless, we hope the book will offer enough background for all readers to understand new advances as they develop.

2. To discuss the ethical and halachic issues related to genetics. These include techniques used for the prevention of genetic diseases and the mapping of the human genome.

3. To review what are generally known as "Jewish genetic diseases" in that they are most common in those of Jewish descent— both Eastern (Sephardi) and Western (Ashkenazi). In some cases the disease is more common among Jews (e.g., Tay-Sachs). In other cases the disease occurs across ethnicities but certain mutations are more common among Jews (e.g., cystic fibrosis).

4. To review a number of genetic conditions that are not unique to Jews but, because they are common, may well occur in Jewish families. These include Down syndrome, Turner syndrome, Fragile X, Spinal Muscle Atrophy, and Disorders of Sexual Development.

5. To discuss issues involved in raising children with special needs or chronic illness such as those that can occur for genetic reasons. For all conditions, we include organizations available to support those families living with these conditions.

6. To discuss ethical and halachic aspects of nonmedical uses of genetics. These include the use of genetics in legal contexts, such as DNA testing for paternity, and research in fields such as Jewish history.

Section I:
The Science and Ethics of Genetics

Introduction to Genetics

Penina Dienstag[1] and Deena Zimmerman

It is not possible to comprehensively address genetics in a book this size—even basic genetics has numerous textbooks devoted to it. However, the purpose of this chapter is to provide the information needed to understand the concepts of genetic disease and testing that will be addressed in subsequent chapters.

Genetics is the study of heredity. Over time, the study of genetics has progressed from observation of traits and diseases to the study of cells and their components. A **cell** is the basic unit of life. It is a living organism that is capable of self-replication and carrying out basic functions of life. Today, science recognizes two kinds of organisms, prokaryotes and eukaryotes. Eukaryotes, including humans, are those organisms whose cells have a membrane surrounding their nucleus, a discrete area where the cell's genetic material is found. Humans are made up of billions of eukaryotic cells and each of these cells (apart from the egg or sperm cell) contains a complete copy of all of an individual's genetic material. The complete genetic material is known as the **genome**.

Genetic information is found in the cell's **DNA**. DNA, short for *deoxyribonucleic acid*, contains the information for reproducing the cell and for carrying out the functions necessary for existence. DNA is a long strand composed of molecular subunits, called **nucleotides**, each of which includes a sugar, a phosphate, and a nitrogenous base. Within the nucleus of a eukaryotic cell, DNA is found in the form of a double helix—two strands wrapped around each other. A double helix resembles a circular staircase. In the DNA "staircase," the sugar and phosphates form the banister and each stair is composed of two nitrogenous bases bonded together in the middle. The nitrogenous bases pair off in a specific manner. Adenine (or A for short) pairs with thymine (T), and guanine (G) pairs with cytosine (C).

3

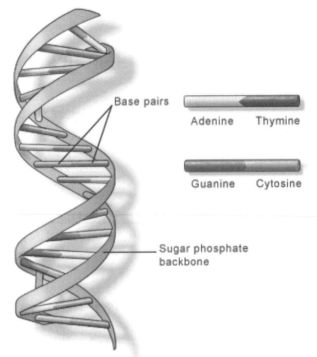

Base pairs

Adenine   Thymine

Guanine   Cytosine

Sugar phosphate
backbone

2 U.S. National Library of Medicine

The double Helix

³   Guanine   Cytosine   Adenine   Thymine

Base Pairs

Eukaryotes also have other "**organelles**," specialized structures dedicated to a specific function. They are located in the part of the cell outside
of the nucleus, known as the **cytoplasm**. One such organelle is the **mito-
chondrion**, which provides the energy for cellular functions. The mitochondria have their own ring-shaped DNA.

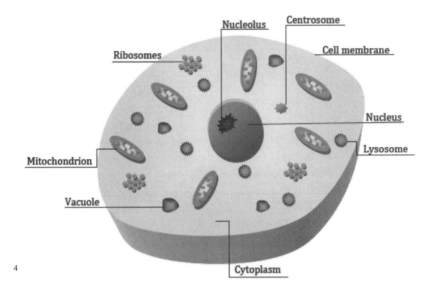

Organelles

Within yet another organelle, the **ribosome,** proteins are formed. A molecule known as ribonucleic acid or **RNA** brings the DNA's instructions for making these proteins to the cytoplasm. RNA is similar in structure to DNA; however, uracil (U) is substituted for thymine. An RNA strand is formed when the two strands of DNA partially uncoil, allowing the individual RNA nucleotides to match up with the exposed DNA nucleotides. A on the DNA matches up with U of the RNA, T of the DNA matches with A of the RNA, and G and C match with each other. The process of writing the DNA message in the molecules of RNA is known as **transcription**. Before leaving the nucleus, the regions of RNA that will not be used for the protein are removed and the mature RNA is spliced together and "capped" and "tailed." The capping and tailing is believed to prevent the degradation and thus promote the stability of the RNA molecule. When transcription is complete, the form of RNA that results, known as messenger RNA, or **mRNA**, leaves the nucleus to carry the message to the cytoplasm, where it lines up on the ribosome.

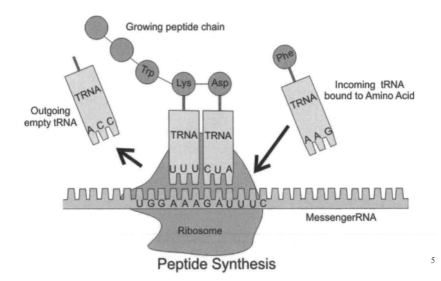

Peptide Synthesis [5]

Another form of RNA, known as transfer RNA or **tRNA**, is found in the cytoplasm. **The tRNA molecule includes a set of three nucleotides, called the anticodon, attached to an amino acid.** Each anticodon recognizes a complementary group of three nucleotides in the mRNA strand, called the **codon**. The tRNA matches up to the mRNA, with each A matching a U and each G matching a C. As the tRNA anticodons line up, the amino acids line up as well. When the process is complete, the amino acids are joined together to form a protein. Creating the proteins from the message of RNA is known as **translation**.

Through the combination of transcription and translation, the order of nucleotide bases in the DNA dictates the order of amino acids of proteins. For example, the codon ACT in the DNA is transcribed as UGA in the mRNA. This matches up with the tRNA anticodon ACU, which carries the amino acid threonine. Thus, wherever the codon ACT appears in the DNA, the amino acid threonine will appear in the final protein.

Other areas of the genetic material aside from the regions that code for proteins can be important to the expression of the protein. For example, if there is a need for a larger amount of an enzyme, a signal can increase or decrease its production; these are known as "enhancer" regions. They don't need to be located near the actual gene, but they are necessary for proper cellular function. Without a properly coded enhancer region, the right amount of proteins will not be available for cell needs.

A progression of codons that has a specific meaning (such as the code for a particular protein) is known as a coding region. A **gene** is that portion of the DNA that codes for a specific trait.[6] A person's genetic makeup for a specific gene is known as the **genotype**. An effect of the genetic makeup that can be seen or measured is known as the **phenotype**. Thus, to use a simplified example, eye color depends on the "B" gene. Brown (B) is dominant over blue (b). Therefore, someone who inherits two b genes will have blue eyes. Someone who inherits two B genes will have brown eyes. Someone who gets one B gene and one b gene will also have brown eyes, because brown is dominant. Therefore, someone who has brown eyes (the phenotype) can have two different genotypes, either BB or Bb.

DNA can suffer from wear and tear. Environmental factors such as radiation and certain chemicals can damage DNA. The cell has a built-in repair system to correct such damage, but this system is not foolproof and different types of errors can creep in. Errors in DNA can lead to errors in the protein that is produced at the end of translation. Many of these proteins have important functions in the cell, such as being part of the cell structure or functioning as **enzymes**, substances that enable processes in the cell to occur. The linear order of amino acids in a protein is not the only aspect that is important. The three-dimensional structure, determined by the way the protein folds, is also needed for proper function. Part of this three-dimensional structure is due to the order of the amino acids, but sometimes the structure can be affected by genes separate from those that code for amino acid composition. Therefore, a small mistake in the DNA can lead to a mistake in an enzyme and have significant impact on cellular function.

There are a number of types of possible mistakes. As explained above, a group of three nucleotide bases codes indirectly for a particular amino acid. Each group of three bases is known as a **codon**. There are 64 possible codons (4x4x4) and only 20 amino acids. Therefore, as shown in table 1, more than one codon can code for the same amino acid. Furthermore, certain codons have other meanings. For example, codons that mean "stop translating" are known as stop codons. The triplet ATG, when it appears in certain locations, means to begin translation. In this situation it is known as the initiation codon.

Amino Acid	Three-Letter Abbreviation	One-Letter Abbreviation	DNA Codons
Alanine	Ala	A	GCT, GCC,GCA,GCG
Arginine	Arg	R	CGT, CGC,CGA,CGG,AGA,AGG
Asparagine	Asn	N	AAT, AAC
Aspartic acid	Asp	D	GAT, GAC
Cysteine	Cys	C	TGT, TGG
Glutamic acic	Glu	E	GAA, GAG
Glutamine	Gln	Q	CAA, CAG
Glycine	Gly	G	GGT, GGC, GGA, GGG
Histidine	His	H	CAT, CAC
Isoleucine	Ile	I	ATT, ATC, ATA
Leucine	Leu	L	TTA, TTG, CTT, CTC, CTA, CTG
Lysine	Lys	K	AAA, AAG
Methionine	Met	M	ATG
Phenylalanine	Phe	F	TTT, TTC
Proline	Pro	P	CCT, CCC, CCA, CCG
Serine	Ser	S	TCT, TCC, TCA, TCG, AGT, AGC
Threonine	Thr	T	ACT, ACC, ACA, ACG
Tryptophan	Trp	W	TGG
Tyrosine	Tyr	Y	TAT, TAC
Valine	Val	V	GTT, GTC, GTA, GTG
Start			ATG (also methionine)
Stop			TAA, TGA, TAG

Errors, known as **mutations**, can occur in the process of replication.

In **point mutations**, only one nucleotide is replaced by another. This can lead to a number of consequences:

1) If the new codon also codes for the same amino acid, the change will not affect function. This is known as a **silent mutation**.

2) If the mutation results in the replacement of one amino acid by another, it is known as a **missense mutation**. If the protein continues

to function well, the mutation is known as a **conservative muta-tion.** If, as is more likely to happen, a variant protein is produced that does not work, this mutation is known as a **loss of function mutation.** If the protein produced is more potent (and thus likely to upset the delicate balance in the body) or has new, unexpected functions, this is **a gain of function** mutation.

3) If the code for the amino acid is replaced by a stop codon, then production of the protein will stop. The protein will then be short-er than expected and will generally malfunction.

If DNA nucleotides (usually known as base pairs) are omitted, this is called a **deletion.** If extra nucleotides are added, this is known as an **insertion.** If one or two base pairs (or any number that is not a multiple of three) is added or omitted, then the remaining base pairs will be read dif-ferently. For example, a section CCCACAGCA would normally be read as CCC, ACA, GCA (and thus code for proline, threonine, alanine). If one C is omitted at the beginning, this becomes CCA, CAG, CA which has a completely different meaning (proline, glutamine, nothing). This type of error is known as a **frame shift mutation.**

This background information can help one understand the names that are given to those mutations that cause disease. At times the mutation is described as the error in the DNA. In those cases, the position of the error is noted as well as what happened. Thus, for example, p.448 G>A means that at position 448 of the DNA, guanine is replaced by adenine. At other times, the position of the error in the resulting protein is described. In p.448 G>A described above, the amino acid arginine is replaced by histidine in the resulting protein. Therefore, this mutation is also called R448H. Unfortunately, there is not complete consistency as to which system is used. Therefore, each mutation may be described in a number of ways.[7]

Not all DNA codes for proteins. Those parts of the code that are tran-scribed into mRNA are known as **exons.** Some of the exons give messages such as "start transcribing from here" rather than coding for a specific protein. While it used to be believed that one gene coded for one protein, current knowledge has shown that by starting at different points within the gene (and probably other variations), at times more than one protein can be produced by a single gene. This phenomenon is known as **alternate gene splicing.** Other portions of the genome do not seem to have a specific message to convey. Those portions that are inserted between the exons are known as **introns,** and those between genes are known as **intergenic re-**

gions. While for many years these portions were considered "junk DNA," their importance in regulating gene expression, among other roles, is now being uncovered.

Chromosomes are the structures in which the DNA strands and their associated proteins are organized. In humans, there are 23 pairs of chromosomes. Each chromosome has a "waist" along its length, known as the **centromere**, which divides it into two unequal sections. The longer section is called the long arm and the shorter section is called the short arm.

Each cell contains two copies of each of the chromosomes numbered 1–22, which are called **autosomes**. The 23rd pair is known as **sex chromosomes**. Females have two copies of the X chromosome. Males have one X chromosome and one Y chromosome. A **karyotype**, or chromosome spread, is shown below.

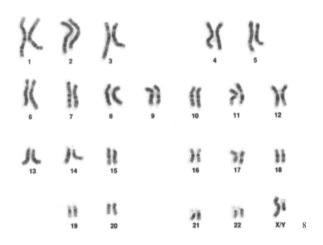

A Karyotype

When cells reproduce, each new cell needs to have the same amount of genetic material as the original cell. To assure this, the original cell first produces a duplicate of all its information. This occurs by a process called DNA replication, in which the DNA strands unwind and then match up with new base pairs to make two identical copies known as **sister chromatids.**

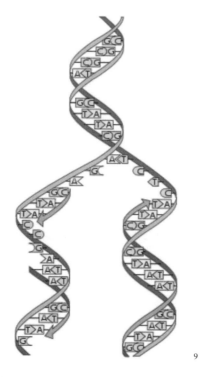

Throughout the life of an organism, cells produce identical copies of themselves for growth and repair and, in the case of single-celled organisms, reproduction. This process, in which genetic material is copied and apportioned evenly between the new cells, is known as **mitosis.**[10] At the end of mitosis, there are two identical daughter cells, each with 46 chromosomes (23 pairs).

Humans reproduce by the union of an egg cell and a sperm cell. During this union, the sperm donates only its genetic material. The cytoplasm of the resulting offspring is obtained entirely from the egg.

If the egg and sperm each had 46 chromosomes, then the resulting embryo would have 92 chromosomes. Therefore, eggs and sperm (known collectively as **gametes**) use a different method of allocating their genetic material, known as **meiosis**.[11] Meiosis involves two cell divisions and results in four cells. Each daughter cell contains only one copy of each of the 23 chromosomes, and thus has half the amount of genetic material of the parent. This condition is called **haploid**.

In the process that makes human male gametes (spermatogenesis), four equal sperm cells are produced.[12] In the process that makes human female gametes (oogenesis), the cytoplasm is divided unequally.[13] As illustrated below, the final result is one mature egg (ovum), which has most of the cytoplasm, and three entities, which contain a nucleus but little cytoplasm, known as polar bodies.

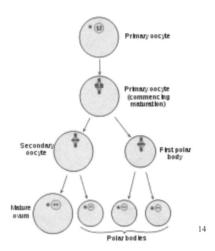

At conception, the haploid gametes fuse and the resulting cell—which will develop into an embryo—once again has the full complement of genetic material. In this situation, known as **diploid**, there are two copies of every gene. In general, one is inherited from the mother and the other from the father. The copy of the gene on each chromosome is known as an **allele**.

At times, cell division does not proceed as smoothly as outlined above. An error called **non-disjunction** can occur if the chromosomes do not separate evenly. One gamete will end up with an extra copy of a particular chromosome, and the other with a missing copy. If the one with the extra copy is fertilized by a normal gamete, the resulting fetus will have three copies of the chromosome in question rather than two. This is known as a **trisomy**. If the cell with the missing copy is fertilized by a normal cell, the resulting fetus will have only one copy of the chromosome in question. This is known as **monosomy**. At times, a portion of one chromosome will somehow find its way onto another chromosome. This process is called **translocation**. If all the genetic material is still present in the cell in a functional manner, this is called a **balanced translocation**. Carriers of this kind of mutation usually are asymptomatic. However, their children may be affected. During meiosis, part of the material may go to one daughter cell and the other to the other daughter cell. Offspring that result from the union with these unbalanced daughter cells can have trisomy or monosomy of the genetic material of part of the chromosome even if the total number of chromosomes is normal. At times, a portion of one chromosome will be cut off; this is known as a **deletion**. Conditions that arise from mistakes in chromosomal number are known as **chromosomal disorders**. A common example is trisomy 21, or Down syndrome.

As discussed above, errors, known as mutations, can also occur in the replication of DNA. When these mutations result in an observable deleterious effect, this can be associated with a **genetic disease, disorder,** or **condition**. Prior to the explosion of knowledge in genetics, it was fairly easy to define genetic diseases. These were either diseases caused by nondisjunction as described above, or **single gene disorders** caused by a mutation in one gene.

Single gene disorders are generally divided into subtypes that reflect their method of inheritance:

a. **Dominant**—these conditions are manifest in offspring even if only one copy of the abnormal gene is inherited.

b. **Recessive**—in order to have the symptoms of a recessive condition, a person has to inherit two defective genes. Carriers of the gene, who have only one copy with the mutation, are healthy.

c. **X linked**—in these conditions, the affected gene is on the X chromosome.

One can calculate the chances for a child inheriting a single gene disorder or being a carrier for each condition.

As described above, after meiosis, each gamete has half the genetic material of the parent. With fertilization, this is joined to the half from the other parent. If one defective copy (indicated by A' in the figure below) is sufficient to cause disease, this is called an **autosomal dominant**

condition. Each child of a parent with such a condition has a 50 percent chance of getting the condition. The other 50 percent do not have the disease and are not carriers.

		Maternal	
		A	A'
Paternal	A	AA	AA'
	A	AA	AA'

In an **autosomal recessive condition**, one needs two copies of the affected gene (shown as a) to have the condition. A person who has only one copy of the affected gene is called a **carrier** and will not be affected by the condition. If a carrier (Aa) has children with a noncarrier (AA), none of the children will have the condition. Each child will have a 50 percent chance of being a carrier.

		Maternal	
		A	a
Paternal	A	AA	Aa
	A	AA	Aa

		Maternal	
		A	a
Paternal	A	AA	Aa
	a	Aa	aa

If two carriers have children, there are three possible outcomes. There is a 50 percent chance of the child being a carrier (Aa), a 25 percent chance the child will not carry the mutation (AA), and a 25 percent chance the child will have the genetic makeup leading to the condition (aa). Having one copy of a recessively inherited gene is known as being **heterozygous** (Aa). Having two copies is known as being **homozygous** (aa).

The proportion of people within a given population who are carriers of an autosomal recessive condition (people who are Aa) is called the **carrier**

frequency. For example, a carrier frequency of 1:20 means that one out of every 20 people in the population carries the mutation. This means that approximately one out of every 400 marriages will be between two carriers. Approximately one-quarter of the children from every such marriage will be affected (aa). Thus, in this population, one would expect one out of every 1,600 children to be affected by the condition.

In X linked disorders, there are different outcomes for male and female offspring. Females have two X chromosomes. Therefore, if they inherit an affected X chromosome (X*), they still generally have one normal X chromosome.[15] Females can be affected if they get an X chromosome bearing the mutation from both parents (X*X*), as then there is no normal X chromosome.

The mother passes on her X chromosomes to both her sons and daughters. If she is a carrier of an X linked condition, her offspring have a 50 percent chance of getting the affected X and a 50 percent chance of getting the normal X. Assuming the father does not himself have the X linked disease, he will give a normal X chromosome to his daughters. Therefore, a girl born to a carrier mother has a 50 percent chance of being a carrier and a 50 percent chance of being completely unaffected.

Males, on the other hand, have one X chromosome (that they inherit from their mother) and one Y chromosome (that they inherit from their father). If the mother is a carrier of an X linked condition, her sons have a 50 percent chance of having the condition and a 50 percent chance of not having the abnormal gene at all.

		Maternal	
		X*	X
Paternal	X	X*X	XX
	Y	X*Y	XY

Because males have only one X chromosome, if there is an affected X, they will have the X linked condition. They cannot be carriers. Fathers who have the abnormal X (X*Y), and thus are affected by the condition, will pass it down to all of their daughters and none of their sons. The daughters will be carriers and the sons will not have the affected gene for the condition.

		Maternal	
		X	X
Paternal	X*	X*X	X*X
	Y	XY	XY

If a woman who is a carrier marries a man who has the condition, each daughter will either have the condition or be a carrier (there is a 50 percent chance of each outcome). Each son will have a 50 percent chance of having the condition.

		Maternal	
		X*	X
Paternal	X*	X*X*	X*X
	Y	X*Y	XY

Conditions that follow these patterns of inheritance are known as Mendelian Disorders in honor of Gregor Mendel, the Austrian monk who elucidated them. Mendelian disorders still show the most common clear associations between genetic makeup and disease. However, it is becoming clear that these are not the only methods of inheritance.

Mitochondria have their own DNA. When the error is in the DNA of the mitochondria rather than the DNA of the nucleus, the resulting disease is known as a **mitochondrial disease**. As only the nuclear component of the sperm cell is involved in fertilization, mitochondria are inherited from one's mother. Therefore, mitochondrial diseases are passed from a mother to her offspring. All of her children, regardless of their gender, will be affected.

Sometimes, inheritance is not as clear cut as it appears from the above explanations. In certain conditions, **some** of those who have the gene will get the disease but others will not. The degree to which those with the gene will get the condition is known as **penetrance**. Thus, if all those with a dominant affected gene or two copies of a recessive gene develop the condition, the gene is said to have **complete penetrance**. If only a portion will develop the condition, this is known as **incomplete penetrance** or **variable** penetrance. For most condition, it does not matter from which parent a genetic mutation is inherited. However, in some conditions it does. This relates to a phenomenon known as **genetic imprinting**.

Recently, it has been realized that mutations in individual genes are not the only factor in causing genetic diseases. The products of many genes interact with each other. A complex array of molecular signals turns specific genes ON or OFF in specific cells at specific times. Mutations in those parts of the gene that affect such regulation are known as **regulatory mutations**. Modifications of the gene by adding methyl groups to the nucleotides (known as methylation) or by changing the DNA packaging proteins called histones (known as histone modification) can alter the effect of a gene. These "outside of the gene" changes are known as **epigenetic phenomena**. At times, genetic diseases are caused not by changes in a particular gene but rather by changes in the number of times the gene is repeated. This phenomenon is known as **copy number variations**.

Not all differences in genes between individuals are considered mutations. Some are just variations on a theme. These are called **polymorphisms**. The A and B genes for blood groups are such an example.[16] These polymorphisms are being studied as markers for genetic differences between individuals in areas such as response to diseases or medications.

The dawning understanding of the complexity of genetic information has led to the evolution of a new field known as **genomics**.[17] Genetics is the study of single genes and their effects. "Genomics" is the study not just of single genes, but of the functions and interactions of all the genes in the genome.[18] The science of genomics rests on direct experimental access to the entire genome, made possible by the mapping of the human genome. It is hoped that this discipline will help us further understand common conditions that "run in families" but that are not inherited in the manners described above. These include **multigenic conditions** and **multifactorial conditions.** In multigenic disorders, damage is required to more than one gene for the condition to arise. This is seen in a number of forms of cancer. In multifactorial conditions there is an interaction of one's genetic makeup with the environment. Thus, for example, high blood pressure runs in families. However, it is more likely to appear in those family members who are obese than in those who exercise and maintain an ideal body weight.

It does seem that the more we learn, the more there is to know. If the writers of the Psalms saw the wonder of Hashem in the enormity of the universe and the distance of the stars, today we can see it on the microscopic level of the human cell and its functions.

1. Penina Dienstag is a fourth-year medical student at the Sackler School of Medicine – New York Program and graduate of Nishmat's Keren Ariel Program.

2. Figure from http://ghr.nlm.nih.gov/handbook/basics/dna

3. Figures from http://en.wikipedia.org/wiki/Base_pair

4. http://www2.le.ac.uk/departments/emfpu/genetics/explained/mitochondrial

5. http://upload.wikimedia.org/wikipedia/commons/0/0f/Peptide_syn.png

6. The term "gene" can actually have a number of meanings. These can include an archive of information, an interchangeable part, the cause of a disease, the information that makes a protein, a unit of development, and a unit of heredity. For further elucidation of this point (and interesting philosophical discussions of genetics) see Ridley, M. The Agile Gene: Nature vs. Nurture, Chapter 9. New York: Harper Collins, 2003.

7. Sometimes there are also differences in how the positions are numbered.

8. http://en.wikipedia.org/wiki/File:NHGRI_human_male_karyotype.png

9. http://en.wikipedia.org/wiki/DNA_replication

10. This process, which takes between one and two hours to complete, proceeds as follows:

In the first stage, called prophase, the chromosomes, which are generally not visible in most of the cell cycle (known as interphase), become visible. The chromosomes are not condensed during interphase as the DNA is being read to be used for cell functioning. During prophase the chromosomes condense and are packaged and coiled. The two sister chromatids join together at the centromere. The nuclear membrane disappears. Spindle fibers (essentially long chains) begin to form and radiate from points at opposite poles of the cell known as centrioles. The spindle fibers will attach to the centromere of each pair of chromatids.

In the next phase, known as metaphase, the chromosomes are in their most condensed and visible form (in fact studies to determine chromosomal abnormalities are usually performed when the cell is in metaphase. When stained, differential uptake of the stain causes what looks like bands to appear. These bands are used to help describe the location on a chromosome). During metaphase, the chromosomes are still paired with their copy sister chromatid. The pairs line up along the center of the cell, known as the equatorial plane. The spindle fibers are beginning to pull the pairs apart from each other at the centromere.

During the next phase, anaphase, the centromeres split and the sister chromatids are pulled apart and moved toward the opposite sides of the cell. These chromosomes should be identical if the copying of the DNA occurred correctly.

In the last phase, telophase, the cell's structures begin to form again in duplicate. Nuclear membranes form around each of the sets of chromosomes. The spindle fibers disappear, and the chromosomes themselves begin to de-condense and to return to their interphase state where they are not visible. Cytokinesis, the division of the cytoplasm, also occurs.

11. Although the names of parts of meiosis are the same as those during mitosis (with the addition of a Roman numeral I to differentiate the two processes), what occurs during certain phases of meiosis is different:

During interphase I, the genetic material is copied just as in mitosis.

In prophase I, the chromosomes condense and become visible. Then a process unique to meiosis, called synapsis, takes place. During synapsis, the pair of similar chromosomes, known as homologous chromosomes, line up exactly. Two chromosomes means there are four chromatids. Bridges form between the homologous chromosomes and there is an exchange of genetic information. These bridges are called chiasmata. The exchange of information is called crossing over. Toward the end of prophase, the groups of four chromatids, known as tetrads, begin to move toward the equatorial plane. The nuclear membrane disappears and a spindle apparatus forms in the cytoplasm.

During the next phase, metaphase I, the attached tetrads are lined up at the equatorial plate with the chiasmata still in place and with the two sister chromatids at opposite sides of the equatorial plane.

In anaphase I, the chiasmata disappear and the homologous chromosomes are separated. The sister chromatids remain paired at their centromeres. When the cells split, 23 chromosomes remain in each cell, although each is still paired with its sister chromatid.

The second DNA division begins with interphase II—in this part of meiosis no DNA replication occurs. In prophase, metaphase, and anaphase II, the process is similar to mitosis. The chromatids line up, the centromeres are pulled apart by the new spindle fibers, and the sister chromatids each move toward opposite sides of the cell. These chromatids are not identical, due to the crossing over that occurred during prophase I. At the end of anaphase II, there is a total of four new cells, each with 23 chromosomes. Due to the crossing over process that occurred in the first division, these four cells are not genetically identical to the original cell that began the process or each other.

12. Spermatogenesis occurs throughout a male's reproductive life.

13. Female gametes are created when the female is in utero. They remain in suspension before meiosis until the onset of ovulation, when some oocytes (egg cells) will undergo the first cell division, known as meiosis I. The second cell division, meiosis II, will only be completed if the oocyte is fertilized.

14. http://en.wikipedia.org/wiki/Polar_body

15. This is not always true, because as part of normal development of all females, the cell uses only one X chromosome and "shuts down" the other. Which X is shut down is a random event. Therefore, if in many cells the normal X is shut down, the female may be affected. However, as it is likely that in many cells it will be the abnormal X that shuts down, females are generally less affected.

16. Blood types are a combination of these genes. Those with type B blood have either one or two copies of B (BB or BO, as the B gene is dominant). Those with

type A have either one or two copies (AA or AO, as A is also dominant to O). Type O means having neither; type AB means having both, as neither A nor B is dominant to the other.

17. McKusick V. A., Ruddle F. H. A new discipline, a new name, a new journal. Genomics 1987;1:1–2.
18. Guttmacher A. E., and Collins F. S. Genomic Medicine—A Primer. N Engl J Med 2002; 347:1512–1520.

What Is the Connection between Judaism and Genetics?

Genetics in Traditional Sources

Already in *Breishit* we encounter the concept of children resembling their parents. For example, the verse used to describe the birth of Shet to Adam states *bidmutu k'tzalmo*—"in his likeness and image"—a phrase that certainly suggests a resemblance between the two.[1] A midrash brought by the Talmud (*Bava Metzia* 87a) cites the facial resemblance of Yitzchak to Avraham as proof of Avraham's parentage of Yitzchak.[2]

For thousands of years humans have been breeding animals and plants for desirable traits. At least one interpretation of Yaakov's actions with Lavan's sheep[3] is that this was a form of selective breeding.[4]

The Talmud demonstrates an understanding of familial tendencies toward specific diseases. In *Yevamot* 64b the Talmud discusses the case of a woman whose sons died after circumcision. The halachic debate is whether one determines that this is a familial tendency after two cases or three. It is clear that the discussion is one of familial tendency, as the debate is followed by a "case report" of four sisters who lived in Tzipori, three of whom had a first son who died after circumcision. The fourth sister then came to Rabbi Shimon ben Gamliel to ask if she had to circumcise her son. It is clear that the reason for the deaths was excessive bleeding, since in the continuation of the debate it states: "There are families whose blood flows and families whose blood clots."[5] The case of the three sisters is quite suggestive of hemophilia, a bleeding disorder known to be an X linked condition and thus carried by females and affecting their sons. In light of modern understanding of a high carrier frequency of deficiency of certain clotting factors in the Jewish community, it is possible that some cases of multiple sons from the same couple might be an early documentation of one of these genetic mutations.[6]

The same talmudic passage also counsels against marrying into a family with multiple cases of epilepsy.[7] This statement is cited as *halacha* by the Rambam[8] and the *Shulchan Aruch*.[9] However, it should be pointed out that it applies only when there are multiple cases in the family. Furthermore, it is likely that with the modern understanding of the treatability of most cases of epilepsy, this *halacha* is not applicable in most cases. This dictum has been expanded in *teshuvot* to include avoiding marriage into other families with genetic illnesses.[10] However, here too, with the greater understanding of how particular diseases are inherited, this dictum needs to be tailored to specific cases where the risk is real, and not taken as a blanket statement to avoid an entire family.

Another injunction to avoid marriages that strengthen the inheritance of certain traits is found in *Bechorot* 45b:

> A tall man should not marry a tall woman lest their child be extremely tall, and a short man should not marry a short woman lest their child be extremely short. A pale person should not marry a pale person lest their child be extremely pale, and a dark person should not marry a dark person lest their child be extremely dark.[11]

While this phrase further demonstrates an understanding of the heritability of certain human traits, Rabbi Dr. Avraham Steinberg points out that no one brings this recommendation as a halachic ruling.[12]

Jews in Modern Genetics

Jews are at the forefront of the prevention of genetic diseases. For example, there has been such a positive response in the Jewish community toward screening for Tay-Sachs disease (TSD) that currently more TSD cases occur in the non-Jewish population than in the Jewish population.[13] For a number of societal reasons, genetic testing has had a much slower uptake in other ethnic groups.[14]

Israel has also been at the forefront in the field of genetics. The in-gathering of Jews from multiple countries to one small country allows for the study of multiple ethnic populations with relative ease.[15] Discoveries regarding "Jewish" genetic diseases have led to the understanding of much genetic information relevant to other ethnic groups as well.[16] At times, this information leads to the mistaken impression that Jews have more genetic diseases than other groups. While some of the impetus for the long list of Mendelian diseases among Jews[17] is that Jews are a relatively small and inbred community, much of it is that this community has been studied in great depth.

---

1. *Breishit* 5:3: וַיְחִי אָדָם שְׁלֹשִׁים וּמְאַת שָׁנָה וַיּוֹלֶד בִּדְמוּתוֹ כְּצַלְמוֹ וַיִּקְרָא אֶת שְׁמוֹ שֵׁת
2. Rashi, in his commentary on *Breishit* 25:19, uses this midrash to interpret the

redundant language "Yitzchak, the son of Avraham; Avraham sired Yitzchak."

3. *Breishit* 30:32.

4. Y. Flicks, Heredity and Environment: Genetics in Jacob's Handling of Laban's Flock, *Techumin*. Alon Shevut, Israel 1982; 3:461–472.

5. איכא משפחה דרפי דמא, ואיכא משפחה דקמיט דמא.

6. See chapter on Factor VII, XII deficiency, and Glanzmann's Thrombasthenia. There are also Jewish families that have combination deficiencies of Factors V and VIII. See U. Seligsohn, Inherited Bleeding Disorders Common in Jews [Hebrew], *Harefuah* 2010; 149:298–303.

Most authors who quote the stories in the Talmud associate both of them with X linked hemophilia (see for example S. A. Shalev, Z. U. Borochosita, J. Zlotogora, cited below). However, it is possible that this is another bleeding disorder that happens to cause death specifically in boys as they are the ones undergoing circumcision.

7. לא ישא אדם אשה לא ממשפחת נכפין ולא ממשפחת מצורעים. This phrase also includes marrying into a family with multiple cases of leprosy—an infectious, not inherited disease. This is an example of how it is difficult at times to differentiate between genetic and environmental causes of familial illness.

8. Rambam, *Hilchot Isurei Biah* 21:30.

9. *Shulchan Aruch, Even HaEzer* 2:7.

10. A. Steinberg *Encyclopedia Refuit Hilchatit*, s.v. *torasha*. Available online at http://www.medethics.org.il/articles/tora/subject35.asp.

11. אמר ר"ל: גבוה לא ישא גבוהית - שמא יצא מהן תורן, ננס לא ישא ננסת - שמא יצא מהם אצבעי, לבן לא ישא לבנה - שמא יצא מהם בוהק, שחור לא ישא שחורה - שמא יצא מהן טפוח.

12. A. Steinberg, *Encyclopedia Refuit Hilchatit*, s.v. *torasha*; see note 18.

13. R. J. Desnick and E. Ross, Lessons Learned from Carrier Screening for TSD. Summary of Population-based Carrier Screening for Single Gene Disorders: Lessons Learned and New Opportunities. Conference held in Rockville, MD. February 6–7, 2008. Proceedings available online at http://www.genome.gov/27026048#1b.

14. K. A. Wailoo, Carrier Screening: Populations, Stigmatization, and Eugenics. Summary of Population-based Carrier Screening for Single Gene Disorders: Lessons Learned and New Opportunities. Conference held in Rockville, MD. February 6–7, 2008. Proceedings available online at http://www.genome.gov/27026048#1b.

15. A review of genetics in Israel can be found in S. A. Shalev, Z. U. Borochosita, and J. Zlotogora, 60 Years of Medical Genetics in Israel. [Hebrew] *Harefuah* 2010; 149:91–94.

16. See, for example, B. S. Coller and S. J. Shattil, The GPIIb/IIIa (integrin α IIbβ3) odyssey: a technology-driven saga of a receptor with twists, turns, and even a bend. *Blood*, 15 October 2008, Vol. 112, No. 8, pp. 3011–3025.

17. http://www.health.gov.il/Download/pages/bookjews2011.pdf.

The Human Genome Project

Penina Dienstag and Deena Zimmerman

A book on genetics would not be complete without discussion of a major genetic endeavor that has in many ways changed the face of medical genetics—the Human Genome Project (HGP).[1] The HGP was a project of the United States government, run jointly by the National Institute of Health (NIH) and Department of Energy (DOE), whose goal was to sequence the entire human genome. The project was conceived in 1988 and formally launched in 1990 to fit into a 15-year time frame and an estimated budget of $3 billion.[2] At the time of the proposal, the complete sequencing of the human genome had never been accomplished. The intent of the project was to make this information freely available to scientists and lay people internationally, in order to promote research and development. The vast public expense was justified by the fear that such information could be kept in the private sector if the research was not first completed in the public domain, and that the progress of science and medicine would in turn be limited.[3]

In 1998 a private company known as Celera Genomics announced that it would finish sequencing the human genome in three years.[4] The stimulus of private competition lead to contributions to the Human Genome Project from other countries such as England, France, Japan, and Israel and to the mapping of the entire genome by the HGP within this time frame.[5]

While the direct sequencing of genes in the Human Genome Project has been very helpful in the search for diseases caused by a single gene mutation, it can be difficult at times to find the location of the specific gene of interest. If one were to think of the genome as a tremendous collection of books whose method of organization is unknown to the prospective reader, one could conceive of the difficulty involved in tracking down many genes. Essentially, in order to find a book (in this case a gene), one might have to read through millions of books because the contents and location of the book are unknown within this "book collection." Therefore other projects were initiated to help catalogue the "library." These include the many resources of the National Center for Biotechnology Information.

The International HapMap[6] project was initiated in October 2002 as an international consortium whose goal was to find common patterns of variation in the human genome and make this information freely available to the public. The intent of the HapMap project is to catalogue SNPs, single nucleotide polymorphisms (changes in single base pairs) within the human genome. Any two humans' genomes differ in only 0.1 percent of nucleotide sites, with the most common variants being SNPs. In general, the closer a variation is to a gene associated with a disease, the more likely it is to be inherited with it. Therefore, individuals who share the variations are more likely to share the disease. If a map of the variations existed, it would help find the location of disease-causing genes. To continue the analogy, if one knows on which shelf a book is located, the book can more easily be found.[7, 8]

The HapMap project works by taking DNA samples from many individuals and mapping single nucleotide variations. In this way, a number of people with a common disease can have DNA samples analyzed. If these people have variants in common, these variations or markers can help identify the area of the gene on the genome.

Reports of the success of this method are beginning to be publicized.[9] One such study found a variation associated with an increased risk of heart attack in African Americans. Another found an association of a variation with different optimal doses of anticoagulant medication (Warfarin).[10] Similar advancements are being used to tailor chemotherapy and asthma drugs on the basis of genetic makeup. This progress would seem to imply the promise of more effective medications with less trial and error.[11, 12]

A project that may serve to enhance the data gleaned in the HapMap project is the Human Genome Diversity Project or HGDP. While the goal of this project is to understand the human genetic family tree and trace its development, some data that are gathered could prove useful medically as well.[13] The study of variations common to different populations, and the creation of maps of what genes tend to be inherited together (linkage maps), can enable the data from the HapMap project to be used more effectively.[14]

A number of additional projects have been initiated. The Thousand Genome Project (TGP) builds on knowledge and technology from the earlier projects. Aims of TGP include a mapping of 1,000 genomes for SNPs occurring at a frequency of 1 percent in the population, as well as copy-number variants, where the genes are the same between people but the number of copies varies. By the time this book is published, there will certainly be more projects, either privately or government sponsored.

From the onset of these endeavors, there were concerns regarding this enterprise. It was feared that knowledge of the DNA makeup of humans would decrease their "humanness." There were concerns that the knowledge could be misused and lead to discrimination in employment and insurance. Religious thinkers raised concerns of man overstepping his boundaries and "playing God." To help address these concerns, an international conference was held in Tokyo and Inuyama City in July 1990. Resulting from this meeting was the Inuyama Declaration—Human Genome Mapping, Genetic Screening and Therapy. This declaration laid down guidelines for ethical use of what was expected to be learned from the Human Genome Project. Furthermore, a significant part of the project, called ELSI, short for the ethical, legal, and social implications, was devoted to investigating the social results of the information gleaned through the Human Genome Project. The results of this element of the project included the proposal of legal mechanisms protecting against breach of privacy and genetic discrimination, oversight of genetic testing, and ensuring that the knowledge gleaned from the project would be incorporated into standard clinical practice.[15]

Many religious thinkers were concerned about man playing the role of God. For example, the University of Notre Dame hosted a conference in October 1994 exploring the humanistic implications of the Human Genome Project, which included a number of papers addressing this issue.[16] The Jewish perspective on the project was not included in this symposium. Interestingly, the concern about man playing God is in general *not* one of the Jewish objections. As elaborated by writers such as Rabbi Dr. Mordechai Halperin, the director of the Dr. Falk Schlesinger Institute for Medical-Halachic Research,[17] and Dr. Fred Rosner, a prolific writer on Jewish medical ethics,[18] Judaism believes that it is the role of man to use the knowledge we are given to improve the world. This approach, however, is not without some dissent.[19]

One story that helps illustrate the Jewish attitude to man-made inventions is found in the *Midrash Tanhuma* (Tazria 5), where a Roman ruler asked Rabbi Akiva: "Which is greater: the works of God or the works of man?" Rabbi Akiva answered that the works of man are greater, and demonstrated this by presenting sheaves of wheat as opposed to baked bread.

As further evidence, the Ramban explains the verse in *Breishit* 2:15 that states that man was placed in the Garden of Eden *leovda u-leshomra* (to work it and to guard it) to mean that man's role is to harness nature to serve his needs.

The permission to intervene in creation is even greater when the goal is to save lives, due to the importance of the imperative to save lives (*pikuach nefesh*). This imperative is derived from a number of sources.[20] There is a further obligation of physicians to take those steps needed to heal.[21] The overall Jewish attitude thus seems to be that traditional Jewish beliefs pose no barrier to scientific advancement in this field.

Rav Meir Soloveichik, admittedly discussing cloning, not necessarily the Human Genome Project directly, raises caution.[22] He cites a story in *Sanhedrin* 75a regarding a man who was consumed by desire for a woman to the point that it was endangering his life. The Sages rule that he must die rather than have any contact with the woman—even if the contact was limited to speaking through a gate, and even if she was unmarried. In the words of R. Soloveichik:

> And as the patient breathed his last, the Rabbis were certain that they had acted rightly; for while every human life is precious beyond measure, even *pikuah nefesh* could not override a larger value, socio-religious in nature—"so that the daughters of Israel not become morally dissolute."... This *sugya* in *Sanhedrin* has, I believe, enormous implications for an Orthodox community attempting to formulate a distinctly Jewish public policy. In deciding whether to support a particular policy, the legalization or prohibition of a practice or procedure, we must consider not only what specific activities are *asur* and *mutar*, what actions are prohibited by the Noahide law or the *Shulhan Arukh,* but what sort of society we are creating, and on what sort of slippery moral slope we might be setting foot.

While there may be a need for some limits, all authors agree that scientific advances in and of themselves are neutral. What is important is how these advances are used. Indications of this approach can be found in the Bible in the story of the Tower of Bavel as related in *Breishit* chapter 11. Verse 3 relates how mankind developed bricks and mortar as building materials. This was the positive application of new technology. The problems began in verse 4, when the same technology was applied for an illicit purpose, building a tower whose purpose, according to aggadic tradition, was to rebel against the heavens.

Time has lent some perspective on the project. The Human Genome Project was completed in 2001 with the sequencing of one haploid copy[23] of the human genome. While this is undoubtedly an impressive accomplishment, the knowledge accrued has also been humbling. At the outset, it was thought it would be possible to have a reference standard of the "normal" human genome to which disease could be compared. It became clear that there is no "one" human genome, since there is a fair amount of variability in many genes that does not cause disease. The 3 billion DNA base pairs turned out to include only 23,000 protein coding genes, only 1.5 percent of the total number of base pairs. Genes have also been shown to overlap and to be affected by other DNA sequences that are not necessarily in near proximity.

Thus the field of genetics has accomplished much, but there is still much more to learn. The Jewish view would be that we pray that all this knowledge be used only for good.

1. J. Buchman, A. R. Carson, D. Chitayat, et al., The cycle of genome-directed medicine. *Genome Medicine* 2009, I:16.

2. M. A. Palladino, *Understanding the Human Genome Project*. San Francisco: Benjamin Cummings, 2002, p.7.

3. F. S. Collins, A. Patrinos, E. Jordan, et al., New Goals for the U.S. Human Genome Project: 1998–2003. *Science* 1998; 282:682–9.

4. Palladino, *Understanding the Human Genome Project*, p.7.

5. A nice review of the international contributions and glossary can be found in Y. Segal, The Human Genome Project, available at http://www.medethics.org.il/db/jme.asp.

6. Short for "Haploid Mapping."

7. The International HapMap Consortium. The International HapMap Project. *Nature* 2003; 426:789–96.

8. M. Andrawiss, First Phase of HapMap Project already helping drug discovery. *Nat Rev Drug Discov.* 2005; 4:947.

9. V. G. Cheung, R. S. Spielman, K. G. Ewens, et al., Mapping Determinant of human gene expression by regional and genome wide association. *Nature* 2005; 437:1365–69.

10. M. Andrawiss, First Phase of HapMap Project already helping drug discovery. *Nat Rev Drug Discov.* 2005; 4:947.

11. S. B. Liggett, Pharmacogenetic applications of the Human Genome Project. *Nature Medicine* 2001; 7:281–92.

12. M. J. Ratain and M. V. Relling, Gazing into a crystal ball—cancer therapy in the post genomic era. *Nature Medicine* 2001; 7:283–5.

13. G. J. van Ommen, The human genome project and the future of diagnostics, treatment and prevention. *J Inherit Metab Dis*. 2002; 25:183–8.

14. L. Luca Cavalli-Sforza. The Human Diversity Genome Diversity Project: past, present, and future. *Nat Rev Genet*. 2005; 6:333–40.

15. F. S. Collins, V. A. McKusick. Implications of the Human Genome Project for Medical Science. *JAMA*. 2001; 285:540–4.

16. The papers presented were published as Sloan, Phillip R. [Ed.], *Controlling our Destinies*. Notre Dame, Ind.: University of Notre Dame Press, 2000.

17. M. Halperin, Human Genome Mapping: A Jewish Perspective. Available at www.daat.ac.il/.

18. F. Rosner, Judaism, Genetic Screening and Genetic Therapy. Available at http://www.jewishvirtuallibrary.org/jsource/Judaism/genetic.html. Accessed Oct. 24, 2010; The Genome Project and Jewish Law: Does the genome project take *imitatio dei* too far—beyond imitating God, to playing God? Available at http://www.myjewishlearning.com/beliefs/Issues/Bioethics/Genetic_Issues/Gene_Therapy_and_Engineering/Genome_Project.shtml.

19. M. Hershler, Genetic engineering in Jewish law, *Halakha u-Refua* 1981; 2:350–53.

20. *Vayikra* 18:5: "And you shall keep my commandments and laws that a person should do and live by them. I am Hashem."

Talmud Bavli *Pesachim* 25a: "When Ravin came he said in the name of Rabbi Yochanan—one can be healed by any means (even if normally prohibited) except idolatry, adultery, and murder."

21. Talmud Bavli *Bava Kama* 85a: "The school of Rabbi Yishmael says, *Verapo yerape* [he shall surely heal; *Shemot* 21:18]— from here we know that permission is given to the physician to heal."

Shulchan Aruch, Yoreh Deah 336:1: "The Torah gave permission to the physician to heal, and this is a mitzvah. It is part of the principle of *pikuach nefesh,* and if he does not do so, it is as if he has committed murder."

22. Meir Soloveichik. Symposium on public policy. *Tradition* 2004; 38:12–18.

23. Each person has two copies of most genes, one inherited from the mother and one from the father. A haploid copy of the genome includes only one copy of each gene. See Introduction to Genetics for more information.

The Ethics of Genetic Testing

Genetic testing includes several types of tests performed to determine hereditary makeup. The tests can be done on various tissues (e.g., blood, fetal cells) depending on their purpose.[1]

Genetic testing can be done for several reasons. These include:

- Confirming diagnosis in a person who has symptoms of a particular condition.
- Testing for genetic diseases before they cause symptoms.
- Testing for increased risk for specific diseases.
- Finding out if a person *might* pass on a disease to their children. This is known as *carrier testing*.
  - If this is done before marriage, it is known as *premarital testing*.
  - If it is done after the couple is married but before conception, it is known as *preconception testing*.
- Finding out if a child has a genetic condition before the child is born.
  - If this is done after conception through in vitro fertilization, but before implantation of the resulting embryo, this is known as *pre-implantation genetic diagnosis*.[2]
  - If it is done while the woman is pregnant, it is known as *prenatal testing*.

Many different laboratory techniques can be used for genetic testing.[3] The appropriate test varies markedly from situation to situation. Therefore, other than standard screening discussed below, it is important to receive genetic counseling before undergoing laboratory tests.

There are two categories of tests for mutations on specific genes; they are known as direct and indirect mutation analysis. It is important to understand the differences between them.

Indirect, or linkage, analysis is done when the location of a gene is known but the gene itself and its function are not, or when the gene is known but there are too many possible mutations to do a direct analysis.[4] In such situations, analysis focuses on genetic variations that are not related to the condition but are found near the gene associated with the condition. These variations are known as markers. DNA from family members is studied to see if they have such markers. If a particular marker is found more often in those with the condition than in those without, one can test for the marker as a proxy for the actual mutation. The logic is that if the person has the marker, he or she is more likely to have the mutant gene. Use of indirect analysis generally requires blood samples from a number of family members, a procedure that raises issues of privacy.

Direct mutation analysis can be used when the gene responsible for the condition has been identified and specific mutations within the gene have been described. It is the preferable method, since it does not require testing of family members and is likely to be more accurate. However, some diseases can be caused by many mutations, not all of which are detected by a particular molecular test. For example, in Northern European Caucasians, 70 percent of cystic fibrosis cases share a mutation of one locus. The rest are caused by one of hundreds of other mutations.

What Are the Halachic Issues with Genetic Testing?

There are many halachic issues raised by genetic testing. The halachic approach can differ according to the purpose and timing of the testing. We will discuss each type of genetic testing separately.

Testing of an Affected Person

Genetic testing whose goal is to confirm the diagnosis of a person already exhibiting specific symptoms is the simplest form of testing to justify halachically. It is included in the overall permission for the physician to heal.[5, 6] For example, if an infant is born with the signs of Down syndrome, it is not a problem to perform a blood test to make sure that this diagnosis is, in fact, correct. An accurate diagnosis can ensure that the child is given the care that is known to best help children with this condition. This same permission applies to the testing that is done routinely for newborns to determine if they have genetically transmitted diseases such as phenylketonuria (PKU). People with PKU are missing the enzyme needed to process the amino acid phenylalanine. The care of people with this condition includes a special diet low in phenylalanine. Not adhering to this diet in childhood can lead to serious developmental delay. Children who keep to this diet and are given proper care can grow and develop normally.[7, 8] Therefore, testing for this condition can be looked upon as lifesaving and thus falls under the mandate of *pikuach nefesh* and would be halachically required.[9]

However, at times the implications of a diagnosis are more complex. The classic example, while not specifically a Jewish genetic disease,[10] is Huntington's disease (HD). Huntington's disease is a degenerative neurological disease that leads to abnormal body movements and progressive dementia with onset in most families from ages 30 to 50. The course is generally slow degeneration and increasing disability over 15 to 20 years.[11] A person who inherits the HD alteration and lives long enough will sooner or later develop the disease, although one cannot know in advance at what age. The alteration that causes HD is dominant, which means that a child needs only one copy of the gene from either parent to develop the disease. Each child of an HD parent thus has a 50 percent chance of inheriting the HD alteration and developing the disease. Therefore, testing the parent will likely raise the question of testing the child. Some who are at risk choose not to take the test. Some who have a parent with the disease elect to be tested to resolve uncertainty about their future. A negative test relieves anxiety and uncertainty. However, what to do about a positive test? On the one hand, the person himself is currently healthy and capable of having children. On the other hand, he faces a significant disease at some point in the future, which he has a 50 percent chance of passing on to each of his children. A typical argument in favor of such testing is that it allows the person to reach a "decision regarding reproduction, financial matters, and career planning."[12] A number of studies have been conducted to see if people whose parents had HD wanted to be tested or not. In these studies, between 40 and 70 percent of people reported that they wished to be tested. However, actual use of testing has been much less, ranging between 10 and 20 percent. A concern related to testing was that those who tested positive might commit suicide or have a reduced quality of life. So far, in fact, this has not turned out to be the case, although the group that chooses to be tested may be self-selected to be more psychologically resilient.[13]

A similar genetic situation exists within the Ashkenazi Jewish community, although it has not been studied as extensively. The LRRK2 gene on the long arm of chromosome 12 has been associated with an increased risk of developing Parkinson's disease (PD), a disease of progressive neurological decline. A particular mutation of this gene, G2019S,[14] has been shown to be significantly more frequent in the Ashkenazi Jewish community. This increased risk is transmitted in an autosomal dominant fashion, so there is a 50 percent chance that the child of someone with the mutation has inherited the mutation and thus the risk. However, not everyone with the mutation will actually develop Parkinson's. Regarding this discovery, researchers state:

> Although testing symptomatic patients may help establish the diagnosis of PD, the value of screening asymptomatic individuals remains questionable until the penetrance and age-dependent risk of this mutation are more accurately assessed, and specific disease prevention or modifying interventions become available.[15]

Concern about what might happen if a person gets medically bad news is a halachic matter.[16, 17] In the words of Dr. Fred Rosner, a pioneer in the field of Jewish medical ethics:

> It is not clear whether Judaism sanctions genetic screening for disease for which no effective treatment yet exists. Judaism is greatly concerned about the emotional burden (*tiruf haddat*) that such knowledge may place upon a person found to have the gene for Huntington's disease in the presymptomatic stage.[18]

The Talmud expresses additional concerns about attempts to predict the future. *Horiot* 12a[19] lists a number of actions that can be performed to predict various outcomes, including one's life expectancy in the upcoming year. There it says that it is best *not* to do them because perhaps a negative outcome will affect one's mood, and this result in itself will have a negative outcome.

Genetic testing can also be used to help predict the course of a condition and thus help in making therapeutic decisions. A current example that is of much relevance to the Jewish population is testing for BRCA mutations.[20] Women who carry one of these mutations are at greatly increased risk of developing breast and ovarian cancer. In light of this possibility, at times interventions such as removal of breasts or ovaries before the onset of cancer may be recommended.[21] Here too, the testing has relevance not only for the woman being tested but for her offspring and siblings as well.

Prenatal Genetic Counseling

The number of genetic conditions that can currently be tested for is astounding. As of this writing about 900 such tests are available, and with the information being gathered from ongoing genetic research, the numbers will only grow. Therefore, genetic testing should ideally begin with individual counseling to determine which conditions are worth testing for.

It is important to realize that not testing for low-risk conditions is not just a way to save money but an important principle in testing. If a condition is reasonably common, then the number of real cases found by screening will be higher than that of false positives (people identified by the test as having the condition who do not actually have it). However, if the condition is rare, then the number of false positives can be greater than the number of true positives.

The National Institutes of Health sums up many of the issues that reproductive genetic testing and counseling present to all women:

> Reproductive genetic testing, counseling and other genetic services can be valuable components in the reproductive health care of women and their families; they can also have negative effects on individuals, on families and on communities. These services have the potential to increase knowledge about possible pregnancy outcomes that may occur if a woman decides to reproduce; to provide reassurance during pregnancy; to enhance the developing relationship between the woman, her expected child and others; to allow a woman an opportunity to choose whether or not to continue a pregnancy in which the expected child has a birth defect or a genetic disorder, and if continuing, to facilitate prenatal or early infant therapy for her expected child, when possible; and to prepare for bearing and rearing a child with a disability. Conversely, these services have the potential to increase anxiety; to place excessive responsibility, blame and guilt on a woman for her pregnancy outcome; to interfere with maternal infant bonding; and to disrupt relationships between a woman, family members and her community.

> The challenge is to provide each woman with an opportunity to have access to desired genetic services in a way that will improve her control over the circumstances of her reproductive life, her pregnancies, childbearing and parenting, within a framework that is sensitive to her needs and values and minimizes the potential for coercion. The value placed on these services by women and their families depends heavily on a mixture of psychological and ethnocultural influences; religious and moral values; and legal and economic constraints that are unique to each woman. In addition, it may be influenced by a woman's perceptions about and

past experience with people with disabilities. As a consequence, women in different circumstances may weigh the merits of reproductive genetic services quite differently. [22]

This consensus statement includes the following principles:

1. Reproductive genetic services should not be used to pursue "eugenic" goals but should be aimed at increasing individuals' control over their own reproductive lives. Therefore, new strategies need to be developed to evaluate the success of such services.
2. Reproductive genetic services should be meticulously voluntary.
3. Reproductive genetic services should be value-sensitive.
4. Standards of care for reproductive genetic services should emphasize genetic information, education, and counseling rather than testing procedure alone.
5. Social, legal, and economic constraints on reproductive genetic services should be removed.
6. Increasing attention focused on the development and utilization of reproductive genetic testing services may further stigmatize individuals affected by a particular disorder or disability.

Trained genetic counselors seek to be culturally and personally sensitive and to let people make their own decisions. Counselors are supposed to present the scientific knowledge available and, without telling clients what to do, present them with options and let them make the decisions that fit with their own value system.[23] This nondirectiveness, however, does not always translate into practice. Counselors are also human, and may find it very hard not to encourage a particular decision, at least subtly.

Other entities that recommend genetic testing sometimes also have specific agendas. For example, a movie clip (last updated January 1, 2006) available on the site of the Israel Ministry of Health[24] clearly states: "It is important to realize that many of the diseases tested for have no cure. Therefore, the only choice is to diagnose early in order to prevent the birth of an affected child." The diseases discussed in this film are Tay-Sachs, familial dysautonomia, and cystic fibrosis. As can be seen in the individual sections on these conditions, there are clear differences between them. One leads to devastating disease and death in early childhood, one to developmental disability and death in the mid-20s, and one, with proper care, can allow one to live until middle age with little functional incapacity. Furthermore, a child born now with a life expectancy of several decades will potentially have the benefits of significant future medical research when he or she reaches that age.

Therefore, it behooves Jewish couples to be aware of the Jewish view on specific genetic tests and to discuss the topic of genetic testing with their halachic authority even before pregnancy. In this way they can enter into counseling sessions with a clearer view of what their own religious values mandate and what options are within their religious parameters. If pretesting genetic counseling is not offered routinely by the couple's health care providers or system, it is even more important to be aware of what standard testing is done by one's health care provider so as to know what the implications of tests are *before* they are done.

Prenatal Testing

Prenatal testing encompasses two kinds of tests: screening tests and diagnostic tests. It is very important to understand the difference between them before undergoing such testing. Screening is a specific form of testing whose goal is to find an illness early in the disease. To be appropriate for *screening*, the condition being screened for should meet the following criteria:

1. It is serious—because screening is otherwise not worth the bother.
2. Treatment given before symptoms develop should be more beneficial than that given after they develop in terms of reducing death or disability.
3. The prevalence of the condition should be high among the population being screened.
4. The test should be simple and accurate.[25]

Balancing the considerations of simple against accurate is part of the challenge of planning screening programs. A positive screening test raises the probability of the person's having the condition; it does not provide an actual diagnosis. Furthermore, screening tests work best for conditions that are common. This is so because screening tests are designed in such a way that a certain amount of false positives and false negatives are tolerated. A test that is expected to pick up 90 percent of actual cases and has a false positive rate of 5 percent is considered quite reasonable.

If 1,000 women were given such screening for a condition that affects 20 percent of the population, the results would be approximately as follows:

230 tests are positive—180 are true positives, 50 are false positives—and 20 are false negatives. Therefore, most of the women with positive tests actually have the condition.

However, for a condition that affects 10 percent of the population, 140 tests are positive—90 are true positives and 50 are false positives—and 10 are false negatives. That means that more than one-third of the women testing positive do not have the condition. And for a condition that affects only 1 percent of the population, 59 tests are positive, of which 9 are true positive and 50 are false positive, and 1 is a false negative. Thus, only about 15 percent of women with positive tests actually have the condition.

Diagnostic tests are meant to give an actual diagnosis. Sometimes a particular technology can be used either as a screening test or as a diagnostic tool. Ultrasound is such an example. It has been found that certain measurements of the neck region of a fetus, known as nuchal folds, are associated with Down syndrome. Therefore, ultrasound can be used as a screening test for Down syndrome. However, this finding on ultrasound does not diagnose Down syndrome; it just indicates a higher likelihood of the condition. A confirmatory diagnostic test is needed. While ultrasound cannot be used to diagnose Down syndrome, it can also be used for the actual diagnosis of a number of birth defects such as the absence of large parts of the brain (anencephaly) or certain congenital heart defects.

Another common screening test is a blood test for a substance known as *alpha fetoprotein* (AFP). If the result is elevated, there is a higher probability than in the general population that the fetus has a neural tube defect—either the skull is open because the brain is not properly formed (anencephaly) or the spinal cord is open (spina bifida). However, many women with an elevated test result are carrying normal children and the elevated result can have a number of other explanations. For example, the mother may be carrying twins, or may be earlier in her pregnancy than was calculated. In such a case the elevated result *did not* diagnose a neural tube defect. It did, however, justify further testing. In that particular case, the next test is most likely to be an ultrasound, which can easily and noninvasively diagnose if the mother is carrying twins. Ultrasound is also likely to give a better idea about actual gestational age. It will also probably identify a large neural tube defect. However, if the ultrasound is normal, the question still has not been fully answered, since smaller neural tube defects can be missed on ultrasound scanning. To search for the presence of such smaller lesions, the next step is often an amniocentesis to determine

the level of AFP in the amniotic sac. This finding is more closely corre-
lated with a neural tube defect than is the AFP level in the blood.

Today an AFP blood test is generally performed together with other
biochemical markers whose role is primarily to screen for Down syndrome, a clinical syndrome of specific physical findings, mild to moderate
mental retardation, and three copies of the 21st chromosome (therefore this
condition is also called *trisomy 21*).[26] The combined blood test, known as
the quadruple test because it tests for four substances,[27] is generally performed at between 14 and 17 weeks of gestation.[28]

The halachic issue regarding the performance of a screening blood
test or ultrasound is what one will do with the information. If the purpose
of the test is to improve the treatment of the child, such as planning the
birth of a child with spina bifida in a tertiary care hospital best suited for
the care of such a child, it would certainly be allowed. On the other hand,
if the ultimate purpose is to abort an imperfect fetus, then serious halachic
concerns are raised, as will be discussed further in the chapter on abortion.
This is why it is important to discuss such testing before it takes place.

To *diagnose* the presence of many genetic diseases before birth, one
needs access to cells from the fetus. Currently, this means undergoing
an invasive procedure to obtain these cells. The two procedures that are
clinically available at present are *chorionic villi sampling* (CVS) and *amniocentesis*. In chorionic villi sampling, cells of the developing placenta,
known as chorionic villi, are removed for testing. This test can be done
either through the cervix (transcervical) or through the abdomen (transabdominal). The *transcervical* procedure is performed by inserting a thin
plastic tube through the vaginal canal and opening the uterus (the cervix) to reach the placenta. The *transabdominal* procedure is performed
by inserting a needle through the abdomen and uterus and into the placenta. Ultrasound is used to help guide both procedures. CVS is generally
performed between 10 and 12 weeks of gestation as measured from the
last menstrual period. In the past, it had been performed from six to eight
weeks, but because of increased finding of defects in limbs of children
born after the procedure when done at this early date,[29] it is generally not
performed this early anymore.

In amniocentesis, a needle is inserted with ultrasound guidance via
the abdomen into the uterus, and a small amount of the fluid surrounding
the fetus (amniotic fluid) is removed. The cells that are shed by the fetus
into this fluid are cultured in the laboratory and tested. Amniocentesis is

also done to test for elevated levels of substances that are indicative of certain genetic diseases. This test is safest when performed in the second trimester.[30]

Invasive tests slightly increase the rate of miscarriages.[31] This increased risk has halachic consequences, since one should not undergo a medically risky procedure without significant justification. In the non-halachic world, the main focus of prenatal invasive testing is to allow the couple to decide whether or not to terminate the pregnancy if the fetus is found to carry any of the defects tested for. However, most halachic authorities will not permit abortion of a fetus due to most genetic abnormalities (discussed further in the chapter on abortion). In this case there is no justification for an invasive procedure that may lead to a miscarriage of the pregnancy. On the other hand, some families may find it easier to be prepared for the birth of an ill child or benefit from continuing a pregnancy without the worry of carrying an affected fetus. Therefore, some halachic authorities will allow invasive prenatal testing even when they would not allow an abortion. Among those who might, under some conditions, allow for pregnancy termination of a child with Down syndrome, some, such as Rav Shlomo Aviner, openly embrace allowing such testing,[32] and others, following the approach of the late Rav Eliezer Waldenberg, advocate such testing only in families already affected by a condition.[33]

While, in theory, abortion might be easier to permit prior to 40 days of gestation (as measured from the time of presumed conception, usually considered to be the night of *mikveh* immersion), the usual timing of invasive tests does not allow for diagnosis fast enough to arrange abortion of an affected fetus prior to 7.5 weeks of gestation.[34] One group reported their experience of providing early CVS for Orthodox Jews who would not have been willing to abort later.[35] The risk of miscarriage after the procedures was twice as great as generally found when CVS is performed later, with no cases of limb defects in their series. The authors state:

> …consistent with the fundamental genetic principle of being non-directive, we believe that informed patients can logically and appropriately choose a riskier path to a medical answer if religious constraints prevent use of a safer path. This is no different than patients choosing not to have an intervention for religious reasons, despite its potential benefit. … To many the only alternative to genetic risk would be to forgo pregnancy altogether. This is unacceptable because childbearing is an important religious dictum in many of the same communities that place constraints on abortion.

We believe it is ethical to offer these patients such procedures, provided proper informed consent is obtained.

A number of techniques have been used to obtain fetal genetic material for evaluation without risk to the fetus in what is known as *noninvasive prenatal diagnosis* (NIPD). The first method attempted involved isolation of fetal nucleated cells circulating in maternal blood. However, the rarity of such cells in maternal blood has limited the practicality of this method.[36] Another method involves the testing of cell-free DNA—in other words, DNA that is not within cells but is floating freely in maternal blood.[37] This method has entered clinical application for the testing of the Rh status of the fetus.[38] It can also be used in the management of carriers of X linked genetic disorders—prenatal diagnosis by chorionic villi sampling could be performed only for male fetuses, thus avoiding the risk of fetal loss for female fetuses.[39] Reducing risk would be a positive development from a halachic perspective. However, if the final result of the testing is to lead to abortion, it would still be prohibited by many halachic authorities. If the testing could be done very early in pregnancy so that the abortion could be completed within 40 days of *mikveh* use, more halachic authorities might permit it.

Preconception Testing

The purpose of preconception testing is to determine if an already married couple is at risk of genetic diseases before they conceive children. While this procedure can potentially avoid abortion of an already extant fetus, for many genetic diseases the choice facing a couple may be not to have children at all in order to avoid having an affected child. This option is frowned upon by Judaism. Rav J. D. Bleich specifically says, in the context of Tay-Sachs disease, that failure to bear natural children is not a halachically viable alternative.[40] Philosophical basis for this approach can be seen in a story brought in the Talmud (*Berachot* 10a) regarding King Chizkiyahu. *Yeshayahu* 38 relates how the prophet Yeshayahu comes to Chizkiyahu during a serious illness and instructs him to take care of his final affairs since he is going to die. The Talmud then elaborates and recounts the following conversation: Chizkiyahu asks why he will die and is told it is because he did not have children. Chizkiyahu defends his position by stating that he has foreseen that his child will do great evil and thus he wishes to avoid this situation by not having children. Yeshayahu scolds him and tells him that the future is in the hands of God and not man.

Chizkiyahu listens, repents, and lives for an additional 15 years, during which he sires Menashe, one of the most evil kings of the Judean Kingdom. This story is used to support the view that avoiding evil by not having children is not the proper Jewish choice. However, not all authorities agree with Rav Bleich. Rav Yitzchak Zilberstein and Rav Shlomo Zalman Auerbach have ruled that for a family known to be affected with a severe genetic condition for which there is no other choice (such as PGD, as discussed below), the mitzvah of *pru urevu* may not apply.[41]

Preimplantation Genetic Diagnosis

One of the recent advances in medicine that has tremendous potential benefit for those who follow halacha is PGD, or preimplantation genetic diagnosis. In this method, embryos are produced by in vitro fertilization (IVF) and tested for the relevant genetic condition. Embryos without the condition can thus be selected for implantation. This method, while not immune to halachic issues, avoids the difficulties presented by abortion, while at the same time making it possible to avoid the birth of children affected with genetic conditions.[42]

As IVF raises a number of halachic questions, there needs to be justification for undertaking this procedure.[43] An individual decision is needed to determine when this testing is permitted. Rav Yehoshua Neuwirth allows PGD where there is a family history of genetic disease and both parents are known to be carriers. Rav Yosef Shalom Elyashiv allows it if the couple already has one child with the disease.[44]

Premarital Genetic Testing

Avoiding a marriage that can lead to a genetic illness avoids problems of abortion and childless marriages. Therefore, premarital testing is clearly the best option from a halachic standpoint.

There is debate about the best time to do premarital testing. Rabbi Bleich originally recommended testing in childhood.[45] At a later date, he recommended testing in eighth grade.[46] In general medical ethics, however, genetic testing of young children is seen as problematic. The American Academy of Pediatrics feels that testing of children should only be offered when there are immediate medical benefits, such as instituting measures that can prevent the disease, delay its onset, limit its severity, or prevent secondary disabilities, or when there is benefit to another family member and no anticipated harm to the minor. When the results of genetic testing will be used solely for future reproductive decisions or when parents request it and there are no benefits to the child, in most circumstances it should be deferred until the child can request such testing as an autonomous individual who is able to appreciate the emotional and social consequences, as well as the genetic facts, of the results.[47]

Most other halachic authorities follow the example of Rav Moshe Feinstein, who felt that the best time to offer such testing is when both members of the couple are old enough to be contemplating marriage.[48] With the current rate of increase of knowledge of genetic mutations, another advantage of testing later is that new genes are likely to be discovered between the time the child is in eighth grade and the time he or she is ready to contemplate marriage. It is best to do such testing before a dating couple has formed an emotional bond. In those segments of the Jewish community where marriages are arranged, this is relatively easy. For this community, the Dor Yesharim organization has provided a very important service.[49] For example, a study of births between 1986 and 1992 found that no children with Tay-Sachs were born in the ultra-Orthodox community in Israel during that period.[50] Dor Yesharim, however, will perform this testing only before an engagement is announced.[51]

Dor Yesharim began in the ultra-Orthodox community of Ashkenazi Jews in 1986. The first goal of the program was to prevent the marriage of heterozygotes for Tay-Sachs disease. Currently it tests for a number of other conditions inherited in an autosomal recessive fashion: familial dysautonomia, cystic fibrosis, Canavan disease, glycogen storage disease (type 1), Fanconi anemia (type C), Bloom syndrome, Niemann-Pick disease, and Mucolipidosis (type IV). It had started testing for Gaucher disease, but in some cases they ended up identifying not only carriers of the mutation but people who actually had the disease itself (mild cases), so this last test is currently offered only on request.

Dor Yesharim testing is completely anonymous. Samples are identified by code number and a couple is told if they are a suitable match (not both carriers) or not (both carriers). They are not told for what diseases they are carriers or, if a match is approved, if one is a carrier. This arrangement was designed to prevent any stigma associated with carrier status. They also will not test for autosomal dominant conditions, because prevention of carriers' marrying will not prevent the disease. Unfortunately, even with all the precautions built into the system, stigma can still be an issue.[52]

Carrier matching works well in the context of arranged *shidduchim* when there are limited potential mates. However, in the more modern world with open dating practices, multiple members of the opposite gender would have to be asked to be tested. If such testing were universal, this practice would not be a problem, but since this is unfortunately not yet the case, some rabbis, such as Rabbi Yosef Blau of Yeshiva University, recommend open testing.[53] Open testing has the additional benefit of the person knowing what he or she is a carrier for and thus allows more guided genetic advice for their children.

Open testing is available in many locations. Information regarding local testing sites can be obtained via the Chicago Center for Jewish Genetic Disorders or the Victor Centers for Jewish Genetic Diseases.[54] Open testing for a full panel of genetic diseases[55] is more expensive than Dor Yesharim.[56] In Israel, open testing for certain diseases is available through the Department of Health and for others through one's health fund. One should check with one's health fund for the most up-to-date information.

Despite the debates as to the best method of testing, halachic consensus is clearly emerging that *some* testing should be done. In the words of Rabbi Mordechai Willig, "Use either method, but use something." He has also publicly stated that he will not perform the marriage ceremony for a couple that was not tested.[57] It would seem that at present, performance of genetic testing, at least at the premarital stage, may well be a halachic imperative.

Until recently, the main goal of premarital testing was to call off the engagement of couples who are both carriers. With the advent of PGD, however, it is possible for a couple who are both carriers to marry and still have children who are known in advance not to have the genetic condition. It should be remembered, however, that PGD is expensive and requires the couple (especially the woman) to undergo all the stress and risks associated with IVF while practicing contraception at all other times.

It is also important to realize that, as the list of genetic diseases that can be tested for grows, preventing the marriage of couples who both carry a mutation for *any* genetic disease may markedly limit potential marriages. Therefore, one should understand the condition before it is tested for—and that is part of the impetus for the Genetic Diseases section of this book.

Genetic testing has made a major contribution to the diagnosis, treatment, and prevention of diseases. However, it is very important to understand what the testing is being done for and to understand the possible outcomes before one allows oneself to be tested.

1. At times, testing of the chromosomal makeup of cancer cells is performed to determine the best treatment protocol. However, in this book we will focus on genetic testing whose goal is to investigate the hereditary makeup of an individual, existent or future.

2. For more information on this procedure, see the chapter on Artificial Reproductive Technology.

3. Discussed in greater detail in the next chapter.

4. AAP. Committee on Genetics, Molecular genetic testing in pediatric practice: a subject review. *Pediatrics* 2000; 106:1494–97.

5. *Shemot* 21:18–19: "If people fight and one hits the other with a stone or a fist and he does not die but falls ill. If he gets up and walks outside on his stick, the aggressor shall be innocent of murder but he shall pay for his missed work and he shall surely heal [*verapo yerape*]."

   Bava Kama 85a: "The school of Rabbi Yishmael says *verapo yerape*—from here we know that permission is given to the physician to heal."

6. Rambam, *Commentary on the Mishna, Nedarim* 4:4 based on *Devarim* 22:2 to restore lost object.

7. J. V. Poustie and J. Widgoose, Dietary interventions for phenylketonuria. *Cochrane Database of Systematic Reviews 2010*, Issue 1. Art No CD001304 DOI 10/1002/14651858/CD001393.pub 2.

8. S. H. L. Yi and R. H. Singh, Protein substitute for children and adults with phenylketonuria. *Cochrane Database of Systematic Reviews* 2009, Issue 4. Art No CD004731/ DOI 10/1002/14651858/CD004731.pub 3.

9. In the United States, newborns are now screened for a standard group of conditions in all 50 states.

10. Although present in a Karaite family in Israel; see http://www.health.gov.il/Download/pages/bookjews2011.pdf.

11. http://www.nlm.nih.gov/medlineplus/ency/article/000770.htm. Accessed March 24, 2010.

12. http://rarediseases.info.nih.gov/GARD/Condition/6677/QnA/18858/Huntington_disease.aspx#50. Accessed March 3, 2010.

13. B. Meiser and S. Dunn, Psychological impact of genetic testing for Huntington's disease: an update of the literature. *J Neurol Psychiatry* 200; 69:574–78.

14. Glycine is replaced by serine at position 2109. This leads to an abnormal protein called leucine-rich repeat serine/threonine-protein kinase 2. This protein appears to have a role in the transmission of signals between cells.

15. A. Orr-Urtreger, C. Shifrin, U. Rozovski, S. Rosner, D. Bercovich, T. Gurevich, H. Yagev-More, A. Bar-Shira, and N. Giladi, *Neurology*. The LRRK2 G2019S mutation in Ashkenazi Jews with Parkinson disease: is there a gender effect? 2007 Oct 16; 69 (16):1595–602.

16. Y. Shafran, Telling the truth of his health situation to the patient. Available online at http://www.medethics.org.il/db/asia.asp.

17. S. Glick, Telling the truth to the patient. *Assia* 1994:2. Available online at http://www.daat.ac.il/daat/kitveyet/assia/divuah-2.htm.

18. F. Rosner. Judaism, Genetic Screening and Genetic Therapy. Available online at http://www.jewishvirtuallibrary.org/jsource/Judaism/genetic.html. Accessed November 11, 2004.

19. אמר רבי אמי: האי מאן דבעי לידע אי מסיק שתיה אי לא, ניתלי שרגא בעשרה יומי דבין ראש השנה ליום הכפורים בביתא דלא נשיב זיקא, אי משיך נהוריה נידע דמסיק שתיה. ומאן דבעי למיעבד בעיסקא, ובעי למידע אי מצלח אי לא מצלח, לירבי תרנגולא, אי שמין ושפר מצלח. האי מאן דבעי למיפק [לאורחא], ובעי למידע אי חזר ואתי לביתא אי לא, ניקום בביתא דחברא, אי חזי בבואה דבבואה לידע דהדר ואתי לביתא. ולאו מלתא היא, דלמא חלשא דעתיה ומיתרע מזליה.

20. B. Meiser, K. Tucker, M. Freidlander, K. Barlow-Stewart, E. Lobb, C. Saunders, and G. Mitchell, Genetic counseling and testing for inherited gene mutations in newly diagnosed patients with breast cancer: a review of the existing literature and a proposed research agenda. *Breast Cancer Research* 2008 10:216.

21. See chapter on Genetic Predispositions.

22. NIH Workshop Proceeding. Reproductive genetic testing: impact on women. *Fetal Diagn Ther* 1993; 8:1–246. Available online at www.ncbi.nlm.nih.gov/pmc/articles/PMC1682823/pdf/ajhg00069-0227.pdf.

23. R. J. Botkin, Prenatal screening: professional standards and the limits of parental choice. *Obstet Gynecol* 1990; 75:875–80.

24. http://www.health.gov.il/pages/default.asp?maincat=42&catId=655&PageId=3627.

25. H. C. Hennekins, J. E. Buring, and S. L. Mayrent, *Epidemiology in Medicine*. Boston: Little Brown, 1987, pp. 327–47.

26. See chapter on Down syndrome.

27. Alpha fetoprotein, beta human chorionic gonadotropin, inhibin A, and estriol.

28. This test can be performed up to 22 weeks of gestation. However, the later it is done, the less time is left in which abortion can be performed, since many locations will not allow abortion after 24 weeks of gestation.

29. CDC Chorionic villus sampling and amniocentesis: recommendations for prenatal counseling. MMWR 1995; 44:1–12.

30. ACOG. Committee on Genetics. Chorionic villus sampling. ACOG *Comm Opin* 1995; 160:1–3.

31. Z. Alfirevic, F. Mujezinovic, and K. Sundburg, Amniocentesis and chorionic villus sampling for prenatal diagnosis. *Chochrane Database of Systematic Reviews* 2003, Issue 3. Republished 2009, Issue 2.

32. S. Aviner, Prenatal testing (amniocentesis), *Assia* 1990; 13. Available online at http://www.daat.ac.il/daat/kitveyet/assia/bdikot-2.htm.

33. *Tzitz Eliezer* 14:102.

34. The earliest time of *mikveh* use is the night following 12 (or in some Sephardi communities 11) days from the onset of menses, the date from which gestation is

medically calculated. Twelve days before *mikveh* plus 40 days after *mikveh* is 52 days, or 7.5 weeks.

35. R. J. Wapner, M. K. Evans, G. Davis, V. Weinblatt, S. Moyer, E. L. Krivchenia, and L. G. Jackson. Procedural risks vs. theology: Chorionic villus sampling for Orthodox Jews at less than eight weeks' gestation. *Am J Obstet Gynecol* 2002; 186:1133–36.

36. D. W. Bianchi, J. L. Simpson, L. G. Jackson, S. Elias, W. Hozgreve, M. I. Evans, et al., Fetal gender and aneuploidy detection using fetal cells in maternal blood. Analysis of NIFTYI data. *Prenatal Diagn* 2002; 22; 609–15.

37. Y. M. D. Lo, Noninvasive prenatal detection of fetal chromosomal aneuploidies by maternal plasma nucleic acid analysis; a review of the current state of the art. *BJOG* 2009; 116:152–57.

38. N. D. Avent, RHD genotyping from maternal plasma; guidelines and technical challenges. *Methods Mol Biol.* 2008; 444; 185–201.

39. J. M. Costa, D. Gautier, and A. Benachi, Genetic analysis of the fetus using maternal blood (French). *Gynecol Obstet Fertil* 2004; 32:646–50.

40. J. D. Bleich, *Contemporary Halachic Problems.* New York: Ktav Publishing House, 1977, pp. 109–15.

41. http://www.medethics.org.il/articles/NA2/NishmatAbraham.EH.1.asp.

42. See chapter on Artificial Reproductive Technology.

43. See chapter on Gender Selection for discussion of PGD for that purpose.

44. A. Avraham, Genetic testing and the prevention of diseases. Lecture given at the Einstein Shul on Genetic Testing. Available online at http://www.yutorah.org/lectures/lecture.cfm/713825/Professor_Abraham_S._Abraham/Genetic_Testing_and_the_prevention_of_disease.

45. J. D. Bleich, *Contemporary Halachic Problems*, volume 1. New York: Ktav Publishing House, 1977, pp. 109–15.

46. B. Yosef, Genetic Testing. Lecture at Yeshiva University February 22, 1990. Available online at http://www.yutorah.org/lectures/lecture.cfm/711492/Rabbi_Yosef_Blau/Genetic_Testing.

47. AAP Committee on Bioethics. Ethical Issues with Genetic Testing in Pediatrics, *Pediatrics*, Vol. 107, No. 6, June 2001, pp. 1451–55. Available online at http://aappolicy.aappublications.org/cgi/content/full/pediatrics;107/6/1451.

48. *Iggrot Moshe, Even HaEzer* 4:10.

49. Dor Yesharim is an organization that arranges genetic testing in the Orthodox community at subsidized rates. Information as to international locations can be obtained via the New York office at **(718) 384-6060.**

50. E. Broide, M. Ziegler, J. Eckstein, and G. Bach. Screening for carriers of Tay-Sachs disease in the ultraorthodox Ashkenazi Jewish community in Israel. *Am J Med Genetics* 1993 47: 213–15.

51. This restriction is to prevent word getting out about a problem in either member of the couple and halachic concerns about breaking off an engagement.

52. A. E. Raz and Y. Vizner, Carrier matching and collective socialization in community genetics: Dor Yeshorim and the reinforcement of stigma. *Social Science & Medicine* 67 (2008), 1361–69.
53. Blau, Yosef, Genetic Testing. Lecture at Yeshiva University, February 22, 1990. Available online at http://www.yutorah.org/lectures/lecture.cfm/711492/ Rabbi_Yosef_Blau/Genetic_Testing.
54. The Victor Centers for Jewish Genetic Diseases National Coordinating Office 5501 Old York Road, Levy 2 West
Philadelphia, PA 19141
Phone: (877) 401-1093
Internet: www.victorcenters.org
55. Estimated at $4,000 in the United States in the absence of insurance coverage, which can vary. See Toby Tabachnick, "Cost, coverage remain hurdles to standard genetic testing." *Jewish Chronicle* September 29, 2010. Available online at http://www.thejewishchronicle.net/view/full_story/9705215/article-Cost--coverage-remain-hurdles-to-standard-genetic-testing. Accessed March 13, 2011.
56. Currently about $200 for the Dor Yesharim panel.
57. M. I. Willig, Jewish gene: genetic screening and the prevention of diseases. Lecture at Yeshiva University, March 21, 2006. Available online at http://www. yutorah.com/lectures/lecture.cfm/714313/Rabbi_Mordechai_I._Willig/Jewish_ Gene:_Genetic_Screening_and_the_Prevention_of_Diseases.

The Science of Genetic Testing

Nicole Schreiber-Agus, PhD[1]

With recent advances in gene discovery, disease characterization, and technology, it has become possible to test individuals for specific changes in their genes or in the RNA or protein products of genes.[2] Very often a directed approach is used whereby one can assess a specific gene, and possibly even common mutations in that gene. This type of testing works well for diseases that result from changes within a single gene (*monogenic diseases*, e.g., the beta-Hexosaminidase A [*HEXA*] gene for Tay-Sachs disease). However, many disorders result from simultaneous changes in multiple genes and/or from interactions between genetic changes and environmental effects (*multigenic/polygenic* or *multifactorial conditions*, such as cancer, autism, or diabetes). Genetic testing for these is more challenging but could become more common in the near future.

When, Why, and How Is Genetic Testing Done?

Genetic testing can be performed at all stages of an individual's lifetime—from prenatal (including preimplantation) to newborn (neonatal) to childhood to adult (and even deceased). It is important to remember that genetic information is complex and must be considered in relation to an individual's ethnicity, family history, lifestyle, and overall health. Beyond these, psychological, religious, social, ethical, legal, and financial issues often come into play when genetic tests are considered; many of these aspects are covered in other chapters of this book. Finally, the decision as to whether and when to be tested is ultimately a personal choice.

Testing is often performed when there is a health issue in a symptomatic individual or in the family. The *diagnostic* tests used may help to confirm or fine-tune a physician's clinical suspicions or, alternatively, to rule out possibilities. Other types of tests are for more *predictive* purposes, to provide insight into the likelihood of disease development in the future. Once a given family member has informative results from genetic testing, his/her first-degree relatives may opt for similar types of tests if the changes detected are hereditary (this kind of testing of blood relatives is also known as *cascade testing*). Knowledge of a genetic issue running in a family can also allow for *prenatal testing* or *preimplantation genetic diagnosis* (see below) to determine the health status of the fetus/embryo. Prenatal testing can also be employed when a health issue is suspected in the fetus on the basis of ultrasound or other clinical findings; these issues could result from inherited alterations or could have arisen spontaneously (also called *de novo*).

Additionally, testing is performed for *screening* purposes on distinct age groups or populations. For example, maternal serum screening in the prenatal period is performed to detect fetal issues such as Down syndrome and open neural tube defects. In the newborn nursery, metabolic and genetic testing is done on all infants as a public health effort so as to allow early detection and intervention for debilitating and/or fatal disorders. *Population-based carrier screening* for single-gene disorders is performed at the preconception (or even premarital) stage to determine risks of having an affected child and to allow for discussion of family planning options. Medical professional bodies offer guidelines as to what tests should be performed on a given population.[3] It is important to note that these guidelines are routinely updated with respect to types of diseases and types of changes that are tested. Accordingly, additional tests may need to be performed with each pregnancy so as to keep the recommended panel current.

Genetic tests are used in the cancer realm, both to identify hereditary cancer syndromes running in families (*germline* mutations) and to determine what changes may have been acquired over time (*somatic* mutations) in tumors. They can also be helpful in classifying tumor types and guiding treatments. In the field of *pharmacogenomics*, testing is done to assess whether an individual's genetic variations may lead to adverse effects or lack of responsiveness to a therapeutic drug, or alternatively may dictate dosage. Genetic testing also is employed in association with tissue transplantations to help identify appropriate organ donors to ensure the best chances of success. Finally, genetic tests are used for other purposes as well, including for parentage determination, zygosity testing on twins, ancestry testing, forensic identification, infectious disease classification, and others; some of these are covered in the chapter titled "Nonmedical Uses of Genetics."

For the most part, genetic testing should be ordered by a physician.[4] The reason for the testing process should be explained to the individual, either by the primary physician, by a *medical geneticist* to whom one was referred, or by a *genetic counselor*—someone who is trained in medical genetics as well as patient counseling, who can serve as a link between physicians and patients. Since family history is a main risk factor for genetic disease, these professionals will often draw a *pedigree*—a family tree showing genetic relationships and medical history. The individual should understand both the test itself and its ramifications, to a degree where he/she can make an informed decision about whether or not to proceed. This process of educating the individual and obtaining permission for the test is known as *informed consent*. Factors to consider include whether the results of the test will be medically actionable and/or will have personal utility (e.g., can the results have implications for intervention or treatment, can they be important for life/reproductive planning, can they change behaviors or lifestyles, etc.).

Assuming that the decision is to proceed, the samples (see next section) are sent to specialized *clinical laboratories*,[5] where the actual tests are performed within a specified turn-around time that can be highly variable. Clinical laboratories are service laboratories and should be differentiated from research laboratories, which focus more on scientific discovery, disease gene identification, and test development. The results of the tests and their interpretation also should be communicated by a physician (provider) or genetic counselor, and where possible, an individual should retain records of those tests/results.

The types of results that can be obtained from genetic tests vary according to the basis for ordering the test and to the type of test performed. A positive result from a diagnostic, prenatal, or newborn screening test may indicate that the condition/disease itself is present. A positive result from a predictive test may indicate that an individual certainly will develop a disease in the future (they are now *presymptomatic*) or, alternatively, may be at increased likelihood of developing the disease (they are *predisposed/susceptible*). However, in the case of the presymptomatic testing, the results do not provide insight as to the likely age of onset, disease course, or severity. With respect to susceptibility testing, a positive result is not a guarantee of one's developing the disease, and it may lead to unnecessary measures and increased anxiety. It is important to remember that positive results not only affect the individual who was tested, but also can implicate blood relatives and future offspring. Genetics professionals are experienced in providing support, guidance, and resources for the family as a whole.

Negative results from diagnostic testing may be helpful in ruling out certain possibilities but also can create the need for additional testing in symptomatic individuals. Negative results from predictive testing may allay anxiety but may also lead people to overrate the benefits of this result (e.g., they may adopt more lax lifestyles). It is also important to realize that the results of genetic testing are never 100 percent guaranteed, and there are built-in disclaimers. Aside from errors that can occur due to laboratory mix-ups or faulty reporting, there is a range of sensitivities/detection abilities of tests that can lead to false negatives. Genetics professionals often address this issue by introducing the concept of *residual risk* after a negative test result. Finally, results can also be uninformative or inconclusive because of technical or biological factors.

Recently a new market has emerged that is known as *direct-to-consumer* (DTC) genetic testing. DTC tests can be medical or nonmedical[6] in nature and are promoted to individuals via the media or internet. The consumer's samples (such as cheek swabs) usually are sent to the associated laboratory (that may or may not be accredited) by mail, and results often are communicated by telephone. Accordingly, the process of educating the individual on the test procedure, its benefits, and its ramifications may be compromised, and the interpretation of the results may be misunderstood. Beyond this problem, many of the marketed tests have not been assessed properly for safety and accuracy. While this type of testing has proven attractive to some consumers, it is currently under scrutiny by the Food and Drug Administration.[7] Use of such tests is not recommended until there is proper oversight of the accuracy of the tests and assurance of appropriate counseling.

Specimens Used for the Tests

Genetic testing usually requires DNA[8] from body tissues or fluids for assessment of genetic, *genomic*,[9] or *epigenetic* (a level superimposed upon the genetic/genomic levels; see more below) changes. For some tests, an individual's RNA or protein is assessed in addition to or as an alternative to the DNA, and these types of tests also fall into the overall realm of genetic testing. DNA, RNA, and protein can be found in all human cells, and for some tests any cell type will be an acceptable choice. In children and adults, blood is used as a common source because it is easy to obtain, dispensable, and cell-rich. In looking for inherited changes on the DNA level, other sources of cells can be used, including cheek swabs, saliva, urine, and hair. Sometimes the choice of the specimen relates to the health issue at hand; for instance, in a cancer situation a piece of the tumor may be used for the analysis.

Additionally, the source of cells could be dictated by the age of the individual. To test in the prenatal stage, fetal cells that have been shed into the amniotic fluid and obtained via *amniocentesis*, or placental cells that are obtained via a procedure known as CVS (for *chorionic villus sampling*), are potential sources. These two procedures fall under the realm of *invasive testing*, since they require the insertion of needles into the uterus. Significant efforts are being expended now to develop *noninvasive prenatal tests* that would involve looking at fetal cells or fetal DNA/RNA in maternal blood.

Testing can also be done on material from very early embryos in conjunction with a procedure known as *preimplantation genetic diagnosis* (PGD) or *preimplantation genetic screening* (PGS). In brief, *in vitro* fertilization is performed and the fertilized embryos are allowed to develop in the laboratory. At a certain time (between day three to five after fertilization), a piece of the embryo or extra-embryonic material is removed and tested for the genetic changes of interest or for genomic changes in general. Embryos that are shown to be healthy are implanted or frozen for future use, while those that are undesirable are discarded or saved for research purposes. This technology circumvents the scenario of having to consider termination of affected fetuses and is discussed further in the chapter on "Artificial Reproductive Technologies and Genetic Diseases."

Specific Types of Tests and Technologies[10]

The technology most relevant to the testing associated with the Jewish genetic diseases described in Section II of this book is known as *genotyping*. Genotyping involves assessing the gene(s) associated with a given disease for mutations such as *nucleotide* changes or small *insertions* or *deletions*, by identifying the *alleles* (gene versions at a specified location) that are present. Sometimes the nature of the suspected mutation is already known from results of previous genetic testing of other family members (*familial mutation*). At other times there are common mutations that are assessed in a given gene(s) for a given disease in a given population.[11] For example, there are three common mutations in the HEXA gene that account for over 95 percent of the Tay-Sachs mutations in the Ashkenazi Jewish population. Testing for 10 common mutations in the MEFV gene can identify 80 percent of Iraqi carriers and 95 percent of North African carriers of Familial Mediterranean Fever. All of the preceding examples would employ *targeted mutation analysis*, since the gene(s) is known, and specific mutation(s) in that gene(s) are being assessed.

Many genetic tests, including genotyping, begin with a technique called PCR—*polymerase chain reaction*—that is performed on isolated DNA from cells.[12] The end goal of PCR is to capture and amplify (make multiple copies of) the target genomic region of interest so that it can be examined in further detail, without complicating the mix with genomic regions that are irrelevant to the test at hand. For genotyping, after the PCR step, a variety of techniques can be employed to differentiate between a mutation being present in one copy (*heterozygous* state), in two copies (*homozygous mutant* state), or not at all (*homozygous normal*). Commonly used techniques for differentiation include *restriction length polymorphism* (RFLP) analysis and *allele-specific primer extension* assays. While these types of techniques were originally developed to look at one mutation in one gene, there are now tests that can assess multiple targeted mutations in a gene or multiple targeted mutations in multiple genes simultaneously (known as a *multiplex assays*). Finally, since PCR is very effective in amplifying regions of interest, even single cells can be used for genetic analysis such as genotyping, and this capability is extremely important for technologies such as preimplantation genetic diagnosis. For some applications, targeted PCRs to amplify regions of interest are often preceded by *whole genome amplification* to generate enough starting material.

Sometimes the specific disease-causing gene/mutations are not known, but instead there are linked *markers* (e.g., sequence polymorphisms or short repeat sequences like *microsatellites*) that are passed down with the disease in the affected members of the family but not the unaffected ones. Then, indirect DNA studies such as *linkage analysis* or *haplotype*[13] *association studies* are used to assess whether an individual has inherited the alterations associated with the disorder in question; samples from several family members are required for this type of analysis.

In certain situations a given gene emerges as a likely candidate but there is no foreknowledge about specific mutations within it that should be assessed. DNA *sequencing* can then be employed to determine the precise order of nucleotides (the sequence) of the gene of interest. Alternatively, alterations in the gene's coding sequence can be roughly identified through a variety of techniques and then precisely determined through focused sequencing (this process is known as *mutation scanning*). With either of these approaches, after comparison to a normal version of the sequence of interest, mutations that have been described previously and character-ized as disease-associated can be uncovered. Complexity in interpretation arises when a novel change is seen, since the clinical significance of that change would be unknown (the change may be disease-causing, may be a benign *polymorphism*, also known as *variant*, or may lie somewhere between those two extremes). This problem in interpretation is becoming more prevalent as technology is moving toward scanning hundreds or thousands of genes simultaneously using targeted or whole genome *arrays* (e.g., SNP—*single nucleotide polymorphism*—arrays) or *next-generation sequencing* approaches.

Changes on the DNA level are not limited to nucleotide changes and small insertions/deletions. Other types include large structural changes where significantly sized regions of chromosomes or entire chromosomes are involved. These types of changes are more commonly referred to as *genomic* (as opposed to genetic) changes or *structural variation*. The classical method of observing chromosomal alterations is called the *karyotype* (chromosomal spread), wherein chromosomes are fixed on slides, stained, and examined. This *cytogenetic* (i.e., chromosomal) technique is used to detect significant abnormalities such as *inversions, translocations, deletions*, and *duplications* in fetuses after amniocentesis or CVS (e.g., the gain of an extra chromosome 21 associated with Down syndrome). A technique known as *fluorescence in situ hybridization* (FISH), where fluorescent probes specific for certain chromosomes/chromosomal regions are *hybridized* to the DNA of fixed cells that are then analyzed under the microscope, allows for the rapid detection of more subtle structural abnormalities. Other techniques exist for the determination of changes in *copy number* (i.e., relative levels) of chromosomal regions including *quantitative*-PCR and *comparative genomic hybridization* (CGH)/array CGH. In addition to uncovering prenatal and postnatal abnormalities, all of these genomic techniques can be employed to classify genomic alterations in cancer. Just as genetic analysis can identify variants of unknown significance, genomic analysis will identify naturally occurring *copy number variants* (CNVs) that are polymorphic between individuals and may not have disease associations.

Recent advances from biomedical research laboratories have uncovered another DNA-associated layer known as the *epigenome* and have opened up the field of *epigenetics*. This layer involves modifications to the DNA nucleotides themselves (e.g., CpG methylation) or to the proteins that are involved in DNA packaging (e.g., histone modification) that lead to changes in gene expression and/or *phenotypes* (i.e., observable traits). These modifications can be inherited or can be acquired in response to environmental signals and then stably maintained. Assessment of the epigenetic layer has been an aspect of the diagnosis of certain cancer types, such as looking at whether tumor suppressor genes are methylated and thereby inactivated. Epigenetic modifications also play a role in *genomic imprinting*, whereby these modifications result in preferential expression of a gene from only one of the two parental alleles. Since deregulation of imprinted genes has been associated with several human disorders, epigenetic testing (such as *methylation analysis*) is employed when those disorders are suspected.

While one generally thinks about genetic testing at the level of genes and DNA, since RNA and protein are the products of gene expression, they need to be included in the realm as well. That is, while we can perform testing to uncover changes on the genetic, genomic, and epigenetic levels, a complete understanding of what those changes mean could require an assessment of whether the genes are being expressed and whether their protein products are fully functional. Techniques employed to look at RNA levels include *reverse-transcriptase* PCR (RT-PCR) and *expression arrays*. Techniques employed on the protein level (also known as *biochemical testing*) include *enzymatic/functional assays, immunohistochemistry, mass spectrometry, Western blotting analysis*, and ELISA assays, to name a few. For example, in Tay-Sachs carrier testing in populations that are not 100 percent Ashkenazi Jewish, it is very helpful to perform enzyme assays to determine the levels of the HEXA enzyme. These protein product-based tests provide a definitive answer as to carrier status, without having to individually assess the 100 or so common and rare mutations that have been described in the HEXA gene.

Finally, it should be noted that while the tests and technologies summarized above are being employed in the clinical laboratory for diagnostic and/or prognostic purposes, the same or similar ones are being used in research efforts to find new disease-associated genes or changes within genes in affected families or in susceptible specific populations. Usually results from the research setting are not communicated to the patient or provider.

The Future of Genetic Testing

Currently there are more than 1,000 genetic disorders for which testing is available. This number is constantly increasing, and health care providers need to continuously update their knowledge about new diseases that become testable. In addition, technology is driving the types of platforms used for testing, and testing methodologies that are capable of providing large amounts of data (e.g., sequencing, arrays, whole genome approaches) will become more routine. Before this happens, the associated costs need to drop, and the ability of medical professionals to interpret and curate the results must improve. There also may be a shift to large-scale testing on the protein level (*proteomics*). The future of genetic tests also will be guided by research findings in *population genetics*, including from *genome wide association studies* that focus on identifying common genetic and genomic variations that contribute to complex diseases like cancer, mental illness, and heart disease.

Ultimately, aside from diagnostic and prognostic applications, genetic testing will converge more with the preventive and therapeutic realms. PGD for medical reasons may become more common, with the caveat that we need to be careful that this and other technologies not be used to test for traits that do not indicate disease. Also personalized medicine will become more of a reality, with treatments tailored according to the underlying genetic cause (some of these exist already, such as the use of herceptin for HER2 positive breast cancers). Finally, genetic testing has enormous implications for the developing field of *gene therapy*, which aims to find ways to cure and prevent genetic disease by replacing defective genes with normal ones.

---

1. Nicole Schreiber-Agus PhD, is the Scientific Director of the Human Genetics Laboratory at Jacobi Medical Center, Bronx, New York. She is also the Scientific Director and Program Liaison for the Program for Jewish Genetic Health at Yeshiva University and the Albert Einstein College of Medicine. Dr. Schreiber-Agus thanks Dr. Susan Gross for her thoughtful review of this chapter.
2. There are numerous published and online resources dedicated to this topic. The reader is directed to the following websites for additional information:
   http://www.ncbi.nlm.nih.gov/projects/GeneTests/static/concepts/conceptsindex.shtml
   http://www.ncbi.nlm.nih.gov/sites/GeneTests/?db=GeneTests
   http://ghr.nlm.nih.gov/handbook/testing?show=all
   http://www.nlm.nih.gov/medlineplus/genetictesting.html and references therein.
3. For example, see http://www.acmg.net/AM/Template.cfm?Section=Practice_Guidelines&Template=/CM/ContentDisplay.cfm&ContentID=2746.
4. An example of an exception could be tissue typing as part of a bone marrow drive.

5. These should be regulated and accredited and can be commercial in nature or based in hospitals/academic centers. Listings of laboratories worldwide that perform clinical testing for different disorders can be found at http://www.ncbi. nlm.nih.gov/sites/GeneTests/lab?db=GeneTests. The Gene Tests website also is an excellent resource for detailed information about specific genetic diseases; see http://www.ncbi.nlm.nih.gov/sites/GeneTests/review?db=GeneTests.

6. For example, some of these DTC tests offer nutritional or behavioral advice based on genetic profile.

7. See http://www.fda.gov/NewsEvents/Testimony/ucm219925.htm for a recent statement from the FDA.

8. Usually the DNA tested is nuclear DNA, but mitochondria have their own genome, and there are associated mitochondrial disorders, so sometimes mitochondrial DNA is tested.

9. The genomic level involves analysis of the *genomes* which includes genes and intergenic regions, thus potentially involving all 3.2 billion base pairs of DNA on 23 pairs of chromosomes.

10. The focus here is to provide an overview of kinds of tests used for the diseases described in Section II of this book. Interested readers are encouraged to read further about the italicized concepts here and in other sections of this chapter at http://www.ncbi.nlm.nih.gov/books/NBK5191/.

11. Mutations that are found more frequently in certain racial/ethnic groups result from a phenomenon called the *founder effect*. This refers to the effect of having a new population begun by a small group of individuals. Any mutations that happen to be present in this small group will be represented in a greater proportion than they would have been in the larger population from which the small group was derived.

12. Some tests do not require PCR as a first step, such as performing Southern blotting for assessment of repeat lengths for Fragile X testing. Here the region of interest is focused upon using a trackable probe that highlights the relevant gene and changes therein as compared to a normal sample.

13. *Haplotypes* are segments of DNA that include closely linked sets of markers that are inherited as a group from one parent.

Genetic Therapeutics

The growing understanding of the underlying genetic causes of diseases is leading to new insights into the treatment of "genetic diseases." At first it was hoped that identification of *the* genetic defect causing a disease would lead directly to *gene therapy*—the ability to fix the underlying genetic defect by removing the defective gene and replacing it with another. This approach was undertaken in 1990 when a working copy of the gene that produces the enzyme adenosine deaminase (ADA) was transferred to the white blood cells through the use of a virus. When these blood cells were injected back into the body of the four-year-old girl from whom they were taken, they in fact produced some of the missing enzyme and helped repair the missing functioning of her immune system.

A setback to gene therapy occurred in 1999, when an 18-year-old boy undergoing gene therapy for the gene to replace the deficiency in a metabolic pathway (ornithine decarboxylase) died four days after treatment. It was felt that he died from an immunological reaction to the virus used to transfer the gene. Then in 2003, seven out of ten patients who underwent gene therapy to treat immunodeficiency developed leukemia. Because of these setbacks, gene therapy is attempted at present only for significant illnesses for which there is no other treatment.

Research is continuing to lead to less dangerous methods of gene therapy. Methods are being tested to inject DNA directly into cells without the use of viruses as an intermediary. Another possible technique is to add a 47th chromosome that would have on it only the genes of interest. All of these methods, however, are still in the experimental stage.

The greater understanding of the mechanisms underlying genetic disease has led to other therapeutic approaches. While replacing the defective gene has been problematic, replacing the missing enzyme has had more success. *Enzyme replacement therapy* is a current reality in a few genetic diseases, including Gaucher disease, which is discussed in this book. If one cannot replace the enzyme, another approach is to lessen the need for the enzyme by reducing the amount of the substance on which it works. *Substrate reduction therapy* is also in clinical practice for the treatment of Gaucher disease. Most enzymes work together with other molecules known as co-factors. At times, giving higher doses of the co-factor can assist the working of a malfunctioning enzyme. This approach has helped in the treatment of some cases of phenylketonuria.

Transfer of working cells has also been done by transplantation from another person who does not have the disease. In the diseases discussed in this book, this is a clinically used therapy for severe thalassemia. Because the best match is often a sibling, such transplantation raises ethical questions. Where bone marrow is transplanted, having a minor child undergo a bone marrow biopsy raises ethical questions regarding the consent of a minor to authorize such a donation.[1] Genetic techniques now allow the creation of new siblings who will be donors through preimplantation selection of embryos that are close matches,[2] raising ethical questions about conceiving a child for this purpose.

Genetic knowledge has also had an impact on the therapeutics for conditions that are not "genetic diseases." Knowing one's genetic makeup provides information regarding susceptibility to disease.[3] Furthermore, different people can react differently to medications based on their genetic makeup. While this has been known for some time, it is now becoming possible to begin to search for markers for this variation. Doing so allows the choice of a medication or dosage that will cure rather than harm. This field is known as *pharmocogenetics* or *pharmacogenomics* and is starting to be used in clinical practice.

It is clear that medicine is only at the beginning of using genetic information for purposes of clinical treatment. It is likely that the current categories of "genetic" and "nongenetic" diseases will soon markedly overlap and that genetics will be incorporated into the treatment of a wide range of medical conditions.

For Further Reading
Centre for Genetic Education. Gene Therapy. http://www.genetics.com. au/pdf/factsheets/fs27.pdf
Human Genome Project Information. Gene Therapy. http://www.ornl.gov/ sci/techresources/Human_Genome/medicine/genetherapy.shtml

---

1. For further discussion of such donations see J. D. Bleich. May tissue donations be compelled? *Contemporary Halachic Problems IV*. New York: Ktav Publishing House, 1995, pp. 287–315.
2. See section on Artificial Reproductive Technology.
3. See chapter on Genetic Predispositions.

Nonmedical Uses of Genetics

Hereditary makeup can be tested for reasons other than identification of disease or the potential for disease in offspring. Genetic knowledge has had forensic[1] and historical implications as well. In this section we will overview some of these implications from a Jewish perspective.

Paternity Testing

Using knowledge of heredity for the purpose of refutation or confirmation of paternity has been done for over a hundred years. The earliest scientific method, starting in the early 20th century, was blood type testing. The ABO blood group was discovered at the turn of that century by Karl Lansteiner. One's blood type is determined by a particular protein, called an antigen, that sits on the surface of red blood cells. Each person receives two genes for blood type, one from each parent. Each gene can be either A (antigen type A), B (antigen type B), or O (no antigen). Four blood types are possible: A, B, AB, and O. Type A is inherited by receiving both genes for type A (AA), or inheriting one gene for type A and one gene for type O (AO). Type B is similar, inheriting BB or BO. Type AB results from inheriting one of each A and B (AB).[2] Type O results from inheriting neither antigen (OO).

Each parent passes on one of his/her two alleles to each child, as illustrated in the table below. The top row and first column represent the allele (gene) passed on by each parent. The white portion of the table shows the blood group of a child from each combination of parental alleles.

Table 1. Blood types of children and alleles received from parents

Parental Alleles	A	B	O
A	A	AB	A
B	AB	B	B
O	A	B	O

One can deduce whether a child may be a possible offspring of a particular parent. For example, if a child has blood type AB and the supposed father is type O, paternity is called into question. If a man has type O and therefore possesses neither the A nor the B gene, he cannot possibly be this child's father. Thus, while knowledge of blood types cannot confirm who the father is, in some cases it can determine who he is not. With testing based on ABO blood groups alone, the evidence can rule out paternity in approximately 30 percent of cases.[3]

Later, additional blood groups were identified. The Rh blood type[4] was discovered in 1939, the Kell blood group[5, 6] in 1946, and the Duffy blood group[7] in 1950. This development helped raise the ability to exclude paternity to 40 percent.

Humans vary in many ways other than their blood groups. In the 1970s the major histocompatibility complex was discovered.[8] This is a complex of genes that code for molecular chains that help the body distinguish "self" from "nonself." Since the nonself is likely to be an invading pathogen, this is part of the body's defense system against diseases. In humans, two parts of this complex[9] are located on chromosome 6. They are called the *Human Leukocyte Antigen* (HLA) genes, because they were first discovered on leukocytes or white blood cells. Each chain[10] has many variations. Since these chains are coded for by different genes, they sort independently and thus *many* different combinations are possible. Since for each gene a person gets one variation (allele) from one parent and one from the other, presence of a chain that is not present in either the presumed mother or the presumed father strongly suggests that another person was involved in the conception of the child. Use of the HLA typing can exclude paternity in up to 80 percent of cases. A combination of blood groups and HLA genes can increase accuracy to up to 99 percent.

Starting in the 1990s, genetic techniques made it possible to directly test DNA.[11] The first technique used was called *Restriction Fragment Length Polymorphism* (RFLP). This technique uses certain enzymes, known as *restriction enzymes*, that will cut DNA molecules in specific locations. The length of the resulting DNA chains varies among people according to the number of repeats of short areas of DNA (known as *variable number tandem repeats* or VNTR) and on the presence or absence of specific locations (known as *restriction sites*). The presence of such sites, and the number of repeats, are traits inherited from one's parents. Therefore, one can search to see if a particular site or number of repeats that are found in the child are also found in the presumed mother or father. While it is possible that an occasional site not present in either parent may arise in a child because of a new mutation, it is quite unlikely that many of these will occur. Therefore, this method is estimated to be 99.96 percent accurate.

The original technique for producing RLFP was accurate but time consuming. However, the same information can now be determined more rapidly through *polymerase chain reactions* (PCR), a technique that can relatively quickly amplify small portions of DNA. This is the usual method for testing for VNTR today.

Paternity has halachic implications in the area of inheritance. A son inherits property from his biological father, unless different arrangements are made while the parents are alive. A question about the use of the "new" technique of blood typing in halachic adjudication in a religious court was asked of Rav Ben Zion Meir Chai Uziel (Israel, 1880–1953).[12] He ruled that it could not be used.[13] His objection was based on a statement in the Talmud in *Niddah* 30a: There are three contributors to the composition of humans—Hashem, the father, and the mother—and the "red" components including blood are contributed by the mother. If the blood is contributed by the mother, then it is not possible to extract information from the blood regarding the father. Others who followed this approach included Rav Eliezer Waldenberg[14] and Rav Ovadia Yosef.[15]

In cases of contradiction between current medical/scientific knowledge and talmudic dictums, therefore, one follows the words of the Talmud. This is in fact one overall approach to such contradiction.[16] It is not, however, the only one. Another approach, following the Rambam (*Moreh Nevuchim* 3:14) and the Tashbeitz (1:163–165), is that the medical dictums found in rabbinic sources are meant to be advice and not divinely given halachic imperatives. Therefore, one may rely on current medical knowledge without taking these statements into consideration. Some bring as proof of this approach that in the Mishneh Torah, the Rambam's codification of Jewish law, medical dictums are not codified. In light of this approach, Rav Yitzchak Herzog, a contemporary of Rav Uziel,[17] felt that the information should be used. Rav Shlomo Zalman Auerbach[18] pointed out that there is an alternate way to understand the talmudic dictum. It could teach that the mother provides the catalyst for production of blood, but not exclusive production.

Another approach to contradictions that allows the use of modern knowledge is that the knowledge was divinely inspired and relevant at that time, but nature has changed so the talmudic statements are no longer accurate. This principle is cited in a number of halachic contexts such as Tosafot in *Moed Katan* 11a (s.v. *kavra*) as *nishtanu hatevaim*.[19] It should also be noted that it is possible for something to be factually true but not fall under a legal definition. Therefore, it is not necessarily a contradiction to believe in the scientific explanation of blood group heredity but state that it is inadmissible in religious court because of different definitions of evidence.

Proof of paternity also has other halachic implications. A child born to a married woman with a man other than her husband is considered a *mamzer* (the product of a strongly prohibited relationship). The halachic status of a *mamzer* prevents marriage with anyone other than another *mamzer* or a convert, and the children born of a *mamzer* will themselves be *mamzerim*. This is a terrible burden and a situation that the *halacha* itself tries to avoid. This effort is seen in a *mishna* in *Eduyot* 8:7, which states that while Eliyahu will come to clarify rabbinic debates, his role is *not* to uncover those families with halachically problematic lineage.[20] The Talmud in *Kiddushin* 71a states that Hashem did a favor to the people of Israel in ensuring that a family whose problematic heritage was hidden will remain hidden. This statement provides precedent for rabbinic courts not using technology that was previously unavailable when the implication would be to uncover *mamzerim*. The need to ignore the evidence became even greater as the technology became more accurate.[21]

Private paternity testing is widely available on the internet. The fact that this can reveal unknown nonpaternity has already been pointed out by the British Human Genetics Committee. Therefore they recommend thinking through the implications of such testing before doing it.[22] The avoidance of uncovering situations of *mamzer* is further reason to avoid self-testing for such genetic information.

Identification of Remains

At times, however, the need to positively identify an individual can have important halachic implications in the prevention of *igun*. A widow is not allowed to remarry until it is proven that her husband is deceased. When someone dies of natural causes in a known place, this can be done by simple identification of the body. However, in cases of homicide or natural disasters, such identification is not always possible. Genetic techniques have allowed forensic science to perform identification based on DNA. A sample is taken from whatever body tissues can be found, and the VNTR can be compared with that of family members in a manner similar to paternity testing. Alternatively, VNTR can be matched with DNA taken from personal items of the deceased.[23] In this case, in contradistinction to questions of paternity, the use of scientific techniques can prevent rather than cause personal tragedy.

This question came to the forefront in the aftermath of the September 11 World Trade Center attack. Many Jewish women lost their husbands[24] under circumstances where body identification was very problematic.[25] Under these circumstances, Rav Shmuel Wosner, Rav Nissim Karelitz, and Rav Yosef Shalom Elyashiv ruled that DNA is admissible together with other corroboratory evidence to determine the identity of a missing husband.[26, 27] Rav Wosner and Rav Karelitz prefer using the technique of matching a sample from the missing person's personal items.

Allowing DNA evidence in *igun* cases while disallowing it in paternity cases seems inconsistent. However, there are halachic grounds for the distinction. The most important is that *halacha* tries to avoid producing a *mamzer* but goes to great lengths to allow a widow to remarry. Thus, for example, witnesses whose testimony is not accepted in most situations are allowed to testify on the demise of a husband. Furthermore, one can sidestep the objection of the talmudic dictum regarding the origin of blood, since DNA information can be obtained from many body tissues, not only blood. Therefore, it makes sense that different criteria are applied in this circumstance.

Jewish History

The study of genetic variation not only allows study of origins of disease, it also allows study of the origins of people. The underlying principle, known as *coalescence*, is that if people share a mutation, they most likely share an ancestor from whom they inherited the mutation.

Using mathematical models, one can trace this mutation backwards until the point where one finds the person from whom they are all descended. This person is known as the *most recent common ancestor* (MRCA). Furthermore, people who share a greater number of mutations at different locations are likely to be more closely related than those who share fewer mutations. A number of findings from these techniques have shed interesting light on Jewish history.

These mutations can be looked for in different kinds of DNA. One approach that simplifies the analysis is to study mitochondrial DNA (mtDNA). *Mitochondria* are *organelles* ("organs" of the cell) that are found in the cell cytoplasm. They possess a small amount of DNA that is separate from the DNA found in the nucleus of the cell. In cell division, this is passed down to the next generation. Sperm cells make no contribution to mtDNA; it is inherited only from one's mother. Therefore, analysis of mitochondrial DNA allows for undiluted analysis of the maternal line.[28] This type of research on about 600 people worldwide has shown clustering of Jewish groups.[29] For example, Iraqi Jews were more likely to have a pattern called U3 and Haplotype J1, and Haplotype I was found more commonly in Bucharian Jews. Another study traced 58.6 percent of the total mtDNA genetic variation of the Caucasian Jews to only one woman and 58.1 percent of the mtDNA variation of the Georgian Jewish community to one woman.[30] Another study traced half of Ashkenazi Jews to four "matriarchs."[31] This finding indicates that Jews are biologically more closely related to each other than to the general population, and thereby supports the claim of a familial basis of Jewry.

The Y chromosome can also be used for analysis. The Y chromosome has large areas of noncoding DNA where mutations can accumulate. The chromosome is passed from father to son without recombination. Therefore, it allows undiluted analysis of the paternal line. This fact was used to try to determine if there was a genetic basis to support the contention that *kohanim* are related to each other by virtue of their common descent from Aharon. In fact, certain findings were more common in those who had a family tradition of being *kohanim*, even from widely separated locations around the globe, than were found in the general population.[32] The findings were less striking for those with a family history of being *leviim*.[33] Study of the Y chromosome also showed a Middle Eastern ancestry for Jewish men around the globe.[34]

The disadvantage of using either mtDNA or the Y chromosome is that it gives only half the picture, maternal or paternal, respectively. Newer techniques of testing the entire genome allow one to see contributions of both parents. Initial studies used HLA testing.[35, 36] Use of whole genome techniques has also supported the contention that Jews have a biological as well as ideological connection.[37, 38] While this may seem obvious to those who believe in the Torah's account of Jewish origin, there have been claims that the Jews are not a people but simply a religion. The science of genetics seems to be more in concert with the more traditional account, of course allowing for a certain amount of conversion and intermarriage.

The genetic mutations that cause disease also illuminate Jewish history. Certain mutations that lead to Parkinson's disease have been found in both North African and Ashkenazi Jews. This finding would further support a Middle Eastern origin for Ashkenazi Jews.[39] At times, the information can provide even more specific information. For example, one of the theories of the origins of Ashkenazi Jews is that they migrated from the Roman Jewish community that began with the destruction of the Second

Temple and exile of the Jews by Rome. In fact, one of the mutations associated with factor XI deficiency has been found both in Ashkenazi and Roman Jews. A different mutation leading to this deficiency has been found in both Ashkenazi and Iraqi Jews, suggesting that this mutation predates the Second Temple exile.[40, 41, 42] Furthermore, mathematical models can be used to calculate the time of origin of the mutation, which is between 1,000 and 2,000 years ago, a dating that is consistent with the historical narrative.[43]

The effects of the Spanish Expulsion also seem to be borne out in the inheritance of disease. A particular genetic makeup is associated with *pemphigus*, a skin disease, in Jews and Spaniards.[44] *Machado Joseph disease* (MJD), a neurological disease named for Antone Joseph, is in many ethnic groups, but occurs primarily in people of Portuguese ancestry. One Brazilian family with the condition claims to be descended from Portuguese Jews in Amsterdam, and another migrated to the United States from an area of Portugal known to be inhabited primarily by Jews who were expelled from Spain in 1492. Taking into account the family names and traditional professions, physical phenotype, and places of residence of the affected families, it is suggested that the original MJD mutation may have arisen among the settlements of Sephardic Jews in northeastern Portugal. Many of the Portuguese families with MJD, both in Portugal and in the United States, bear family names traditionally attributed to the Sephardim.[45] The high incidence of *Creutzfeldt–Jakob disease*, a degenerative neurologic disease, in Jews from Libya has also been explained by the intramarriage of refugees from the Spanish Expulsion;[46] the same mutation in the BRCA1 gene has been found among Hispanic Catholics in New Mexico and among Ashkenazi Jews.[47]

Since the mathematical calculations are based on numerous assumptions, there is still much imprecision in historical dating by this method. However, genetic techniques are providing yet another resource for the study of Jewish history.

---

1. *Forensic* means application of a science to answer questions of interest to the legal system.
2. This is known as *co-dominance*—neither allele is dominant over the other.
3. The percentages here are based on www.paternity-answers.com.
4. A person is either Rh+ or Rh− depending on whether the Rh protein is part of the makeup of his red cell membrane or not. The locus of the associated gene is on the short arm of chromosome 1.

5. This is a more complicated blood group system that is now known to be coded by the KEL gene found on the long arm of chromosome 7. There are many possible variations of the protein that can be produced. However, two of these (K and k or Kell and Cellano) are the most common.

6. The source for the information on blood groups in L. Dean, *Blood Groups and Red Cell Antigens,* NCBI, 2005, is available online at www.ncbi.nlm.nih.gov/bookshelf/br.fcgi?book=rbcantigen.

7. The gene for the Duffy blood group is located on the long arm of chromosome 1.

8. Information regarding the MHC and HLA typing is from C. A. Janeway, P. Travers, M. Walport, and M. J. Shlomchik, *Immunobiology*, 5th ed. *The Immune System in Health and Disease.* New York: Garland Science, 2001. Available online at www.ncbi.nlm.nih.gov/bookshelf/br.fcgi?book=imm.

9. The MHC class I molecules and the alpha and beta chain of the class II molecules.

10. Called HLA-A, HLA-B, HLA-C,HLA-DR, HLA-DP, and JLD-DQ.

11. Source for information on genetic techniques is A. J. F. Griffiths, W. M. Gelbart, J. H. Miller, and R. C. Lewontin, RFLP Mapping. *Modern Genetic Analysis.* New York: W.H. Freeman and Company, 1999. Available online at www.ncbi.nlm.nih.gov/bookshelf/br.fcgi?book=mga.

12. *Shaarei Uziel* 2:40:1:18.

13. For further discussion see C. Jachter, Blood Tests and DNA, Part 1. Rabbi Jachter's Halacha Files 2006:16. Available online at www.koltorah.org/RAVJ/Blood_Tests_and_DNA_1.html.

14. *Tzitz Eliezer* 13:104.

15. *Yabia Omer* 10, *Even HaEzer* 12 and 13.

16. This is the approach of the Rivash (Isaac ben Sheshet Perfet, Spain 1326–1408) Responsa 447.

17. Rav Uziel and Rav Herzog served as the Sephardi and Ashkenazi Chief Rabbis, respectively, under the British Mandate and then were the first to hold these positions in the State of Israel.

18. Cited in *Nishmat Avraham, Even HaEzer* 4:1.

19. For further discussion see E. Friedman, Medicine in the Gemara. Available online at http://koltorah.org/ravj/medicINgemara.htm.

20. See commentary of Rav Ovadia MiBartanura (Italy, Jerusalem late 1400) on this *mishna.*

21. See Jachter C. Blood tests and DNA – Part 2, available at http://w,w.koltorah.org/ravj/Blood_Tests_and_DNA_2.html, and Halperin M., Brautber H., Nelkan D. *Keviat Avhut beamtzaut maarechet tium harikmot hamerkazit Techumin.* 1983, 431–450.

22. www.hgc.gov.uk/Client/Content.asp?ContendId=871.

23. Such as hairs from a hairbrush or saliva from a toothbrush.

24. Many men also lost their wives. However, as marrying a second wife is only prohibited by medieval rabbinic edict, as opposed to the biblical prohibition for women to have two husbands, when permitting a man to remarry the halachic burden of proof for the demise of a wife is less.

25. See also Jachter C. Blood tests and DNA–Part 3, available at http://www.koltorah.org/ravj/Blood_Tests and DNA_3.html.

26. See C. Jachter, The Beit Din of American's Handling of the World Trade Center Agunot. Available online in four parts, at:

- http://www.yutorah.com/lectures/lecture.cfm/736152/Rabbi_Chaim_ Jachter/The_Beth_Din_of_America's_Handling_of_the_World_ Trade_Center_Agunot__Part_One:_Methodology_of_Agunah_Crisis_ Management
- http://www.yutorah.com/lectures/lecture.cfm/736153/Rabbi_Chaim_ Jachter/The_Beth_Din_of_America's_Handling_of_the_World_Trade_ Center_Agunot__Part_Two:_The_Rulings_of_the_Beth_Din_of_ America
- http://www.yutorah.com/lectures/lecture.cfm/736154/Rabbi_Chaim_ Jachter/The_Beth_Din_of_America's_Handling_of_the_World_Trade_ Center_Agunot__Part_Three:_The_Rulings_of_the_Beth_Din_of_ America
- http://www.yutorah.com/lectures/lecture.cfm/736155/Rabbi_Chaim_ Jachter/The_Beth_Din_of_America's_Handling_of_the_World_Trade_ Center_Agunot_-_Part_Four:_

27. *Techumin* 21:123.

28. An interesting book on this topic for the lay public is B. Sykes, *The Seven Daughters of Eve: The Science That Reveals Our Genetic Ancestry.* New York: W.W. Norton, 2001. While the book uses techniques based on the concept of evolution, they need not be in conflict with a belief in the Torah. See, for example, M. Halperin, The laws of evolution and Judaism: Lack of Communication. *Assia*, 2001. Available online at http://www.daat.ac.il/daat/kitveyet/assia_english/halperin2.htm.

29. M. G. Thomas, M. E. Weale, A. L. Jones, et al., Founding Mothers of Jewish Communities: Geographically Separated Jewish Groups Were Independently Founded by Very Few Female Ancestors. *The American Journal of Human Genetics* 2002; 70:1411–20.

30. D. M. Behar, D. Metspalu, T. Kivisild, et al., Counting the Founders: The Matrilineal Genetic Ancestry of the Jewish Diaspora. PLoS ONE 2008; 3: e2062.

31. Behar, Metspalu, Kivisild, et al., The Matrilineal Ancestry of Ashkenazi Jewry: Portrait of a Recent Founder Event. *American Journal of Human Genetics* 2006; 78: 487–97.

32. M. F. Hammer, D. M. Behar, T. M. Karafetl, et al., Extended Y chromosome

haplotypes resolve multiple and unique lineages of the Jewish priesthood. *Human Genetics* 2009; 126 707–17.

33. D. M. Behar, M. G. Thomas, K. Skorecki, et al., Multiple Origins of Ashkenazi Levites: Y Chromosome Evidence for Both Near Eastern and European Ancestries. *American Journal of Human Genetics* 2003; 73:4: 768–79.

34. A. Nebel, D. Filon, B. Brinkmann, et al., The Y Chromosome Pool of Jews as Part of the Genetic Landscape of the Middle East. *American Journal of Human Genetics* 2001; 69: 1095–1112.

35. A. Amar, O. J. Kwon, U. Motro, et al., Molecular analysis of HLA class II polymorphisms among different ethnic groups in Israel. *Human Immunology* 1999; 60: 723–30.

36. J. Martinez-Laso, E. Gazit, E. Gomez-Casado, et al., HLA DR and DQ polymorphism in Ashkenazi and non-Ashkenazi Jews: comparison with other Mediterraneans. *Tissue Antigens* 1996; 47: 63–71.

37. D. M. Behar, B. Yunusbayev, M. Metspalu, et al., The genome-wide structure of the Jewish people. *Nature*, published online June 9, 2010.

38. G. Atzmon, L. Hao, I. Pe'er, et al., Abraham's children in the Genome Era: Major Jewish diaspora populations comprise distinct genetic clusters with shared Middle Eastern ancestry. *American Journal of Human Genetics* (in press, June 2010). Published online June 3, 2010.

39. C. P. Zabetian, C. M. Hutter, D. Yearout, et al., LRRK2 G2019S in families with Parkinson disease who originated from Europe and the Middle East: evidence of two distinct founding events beginning two millennia ago. *American Journal of Human Genetics* 2006; 79:752–58.

40. D. B. Goldstein, D. E. Reich, N. Bradman, et al., Age estimates of two common mutations causing factor XI deficiency: recent genetic drift is not necessary for elevated disease incidence among Ashkenazi Jews. *American Journal of Human Genetics* 1999; 64:1071–75.

41. H. Peretz, A. Mulai, S. Usher, et al., The two common mutations causing factor XI deficiency in Jews stem from distinct founders: one of ancient Middle Eastern origin and another of more recent European origin. *Blood* 1997; 90:7: 2654–59.

42. O. Shpilberg, H. Peretz, A. Zivelin, et al., One of the two common mutations causing factor XI deficiency in Ashkenazi Jews (type II) is also prevalent in Iraqi Jews, who represent the ancient gene pool of Jews. *Blood* 1995; 85: 429–32.

43. C. Oddoux, E. Guillen-Navarro, C. M. Clayton, et al., Genetic Evidence for a Common Origin among Roman Jews and Ashkenazi Jews. *American Journal of Human Genetics* 1997; 61: A207.

44. Y. Loewenthal, Y. Slomov, M. F. Gonzalez-Escribano, et al., Common ancestral origin of pemphigus vulgaris in Jews and Spaniards: a study using microsatellite markers. *Tissue Antigens* 2004: 63:4: 326–34.

45. Y. Rosenberg, Machado Joseph Disease. Jewish Genetic Diseases, available online at http://www.mazornet.com/genetics/machado.htm.
46. R. Colombo, Age and Origin of the *PRNP* E200K Mutation Causing Familial Creutzfeldt-Jacob Disease in Libyan Jews. *American Journal of Human Genetics* 2000 August; 67(2): 528–31.
47. J. Wheelwright, The Secret Jews of San Luis Valley. *Smithsonian Magazine*, October 2008.

Artificial Reproductive Technologies and Genetic Diseases

Matthew Cohen, MD[1]

A recent advance in medicine with tremendous potential benefit for those who follow *halacha* is *preimplantation genetic diagnosis* (PGD). In this procedure, *in vitro fertilization* (IVF) is performed to produce embryos. The embryos are then tested for specific genetic diseases and only those that are healthy are implanted into the mother's uterus. As was discussed in the section on genetic testing, this method, while not immune to halachic issues, avoids the difficulties presented by abortion while making it possible to prevent the birth of children affected with genetic conditions. This section will further discuss this technology and what it can and cannot do at this point in time.

Introduced in 1990 as an experimental procedure,[2, 3] PGD is now becoming an established clinical option in reproductive medicine. A multitude of genetic disorders, be they single gene defects (autosomal recessive, autosomal dominant, or X linked) or chromosomal abnormalities such as translocations, can now be diagnosed in the pre-embryo. The purpose of PGD is to identify affected pre-embryos in patients who are at high risk, thereby significantly increasing their chance of having healthy offspring. PGD offers special advantages not possible with traditional prenatal diagnosis. One is to avoid abortion.

IVF

A prerequisite to PGD is access to the embryo at a very early stage of gestation. Since this cannot be done at present through natural pregnancy, the first requirement for the performance of PGD is that the couple undergo *in vitro fertilization*, or IVF.

Women naturally produce one egg per month under the influence of FSH (*follicle stimulating hormone*). To improve the IVF success rates, women are given extra FSH to obtain many eggs (on average, about 10 to 12). FSH is a natural hormone with no direct side effects; however, the increased size of the ovaries can make marital relations uncomfortable.

Use of FSH can lead to a condition known as *ovarian hyperstimulation syndrome* (OHSS), which can be potentially dangerous. During treatment with FSH (about 10 days) women are monitored very closely, sometimes daily. They will typically be given another medication to prevent early ovulation and another at the end to mature the eggs. All these medications are injections, typically with small needles that are injected just under the skin.

After all this preparation, the eggs are harvested from the ovaries. This procedure requires only a needlestick through the top of the vagina (similar to drawing blood from the arm), but the ovaries are next to parts of the body best left untouched (such as blood vessels and bowel); therefore, the woman is sedated so she does not move or feel pain.[4] The same day the eggs are obtained, they are fertilized with the husband's sperm. The Latin term *in vitro* means "in glass," or in a glass vessel outside the body, and that is why this is known as in vitro fertilization (IVF).

Procurement of a sperm sample raises the halachic issue of *hotza'at zera levatala*—the purposeful expulsion of sperm into anything other than the vaginal canal, or literally "removal of seed for naught." The *Shulchan Aruch* rules that this is a very serious transgression.[5] However, most halachic authorities feel that when the purpose of obtaining the sample is to have children, as would be the case in IVF-PGD, this is not considered "for naught."[6] Furthermore, in general medical practice, these samples are obtained by self-stimulation, and masturbation to produce a semen sample is a serious halachic problem.[7] Rabbis will often prefer that the couple have relations with a condom (with or without a small hole in it). It should be noted that a special, sterile condom needs to be used for this collection and not the ones routinely sold in pharmacies. Other rabbis will allow *coitus interruptus*—starting relations in the usual manner but having ejaculation take place into a collection container.

It should be noted that having relations just prior to the procedure may be physically challenging for the woman because of the enlargement of the ovaries from the medications; therefore the sperm can be obtained a month or two prior to the procedure and frozen for the appropriate time.

Another concern regarding the performance of IVF is Shabbat. Since there is no current life being saved, performance of the needed procedures on or by Jews is problematic. It is often possible to circumvent the need for procedures to be performed on Shabbat by proper timing of administration of medications. Each case should be discussed with both the doctor and the rabbi prior to embarking on the procedure.

There are currently two methods for fertilizing the eggs. One, known as *insemination*, is just putting the sperm (usually a hundred thousand or more) and eggs together in a dish. The other is actually to inject a single sperm directly into the egg; this is known as *intra-cytoplasmic sperm injection*, or ICSI. Regardless of which method is used, the fertilized eggs are known as pre-embryos.

When PGD is performed, all the eggs must be fertilized with ICSI to prevent contamination of the embryo's genetic material with that from other sperm. With insemination, many sperm, sometimes dozens, attach to the *zona pellucida* (essentially, the eggshell), although only one actually enters the egg for fertilization. To obtain the embryonic cell that will be analyzed for PGD, a small catheter is placed through the zona pellucida. A sperm attached to the zona pellucida might inadvertently be collected along with desired cell(s), thereby spoiling the accuracy of the analysis. With ICSI, only a single sperm enters the egg, and the egg is not exposed to other sperm that may cause this problem.

The embryos are kept in an incubator, or warmer, for several days. At this point, genetic analysis may be performed. The type of analysis depends on the condition being screened for.

Single Gene Disorders

If one is screening for a single gene disorder, such as Tay-Sachs disease or cystic fibrosis, the usual technique is *polymerase chain reaction* (PCR). In this technique the genetic material is processed in order to create multiple copies of a small amount of DNA. Even one copy (e.g., the gene in question), can be amplified into thousands or millions of copies that can then be accurately studied.

In a dominant disorder, the presence of only one abnormal gene will transmit the disease. In a recessive disorder, two abnormal copies are required (one from each parent). In an X linked disorder, a male fetus with the abnormal gene will have the disease (a female will be a carrier, but not affected). Over 200 genes have now been successfully screened for with PGD, and the error rate is less than one percent.[8]

Initially, the diseases tested for by this technique were those with early childhood onset. This potential has now expanded to include late onset diseases such as Huntington's disease[9] and predisposition to cancer.[10]

Chromosome Disorders

A different type of analysis is performed when one is screening for an abnormal number of chromosomes. Chromosomal abnormalities are responsible for a substantial proportion of early pregnancy losses, and they increase with maternal age.[11, 12] Searching for chromosomal abnormalities is the most common indication for which PGD is currently performed. This can be either in couples with a history of repeated miscarriages or in older women who want to avoid having a child with Down syndrome but do not want to abort an affected fetus.

The most common technique to screen for chromosomal abnormalities is *fluorescent in-situ hybridization* (FISH). Colored fluorescent probes are developed that will match with and attach themselves to DNA sequences that are found on specific chromosomes. The probes are placed in a solution with the genetic material taken from the embryo. Each probe then attaches itself to the appropriate sequence on the relevant chromosome. After processing, the genetic material to which a probe is attached will light up. For all chromosomes except X and Y only two colored probes should be found. If three are found, the fetus either is nonviable (most chromosomes) or may have significant disorders if born (chromosomes 13, 18, and 21). Three copies of chromosome 21 causes Down syndrome. Each chromosome tested should have a different color probe, but there are a limited number of colors available, so not all the chromosomes can be tested. If one is screening for a known translocation, this is typically not a limiting factor since only a small number of probes are required.

Sex Selection

Occasionally a disorder is known to affect only boys or girls but the exact gene is not known. In these cases FISH can be used to detect either two X chromosomes (a girl) or an X and a Y chromosome (a boy) and only embryos of the desired sex can be selected for use. Sometimes the situation is less clear. For example, certain forms of autism occur far more frequently in boys (4:1), but a girl can still be affected. A family may still desire to choose only female embryos to improve the odds, but prevention of the disorder is not guaranteed. Lupus affects girls more than boys in a 9:1 ratio, and families with a strong history of lupus may therefore select for boys.[13]

Savior Siblings

The cure for certain genetic diseases (as well as for many forms of cancer) is a stem cell transplant. In *stem cell transplantation* (SCT), stem cells are transferred from one person to another. Stem cells are cells that the body uses to produce other cells, primarily blood cells. They are found primarily in the bone marrow. To obtain them from the bone marrow requires a bone marrow biopsy. These cells can also be obtained from the blood found in the umbilical cords of newborns. Since the umbilical cord blood is generally discarded after birth, collection from the cord is a painless procedure.

The hope is that after transplantation, the stem cells will replace the blood cells of the person to whom they are given. In the case of genetic diseases, the hope is that the new cells will then be able to produce the enzymes or perform the functions that are missing because of the genetic defect. This therapy can be a cure for certain conditions such as beta thalassemia (see section on genetic diseases).

The human body has a system to reject foreign substances. It is known as the *human lymphocyte antigen* (HLA) system. The more similar the donor and recipient of a transplant are, the better the chance that the body will not reject the transplant.

Finding a matched donor from the general population requires testing thousands of people to find a match, often without success. Siblings, because they share parental genes, are more likely to be matches. However, IVF followed by PGD selecting an embryo shown to have the desired HLA antigens has the highest chance of success. There have been cases where a child has been conceived for the express purpose of providing a donation for an older sibling. There has been discussion as to the ethics of conceiving a child for this purpose, particularly using advanced technology.

Halachic Permissibility

The halachic permissibility of using PGD depends to a great degree on the purpose for which it is performed. The more lethal the condition being screened for, the more likely it is to be permitted.[14] An individual question needs to be asked for each case.

When (and What) to Examine

In order to perform either PCR or FISH, a cell must be obtained from the embryo in a procedure known as a *biopsy*. This cell dies as it is removed from the embryo. There is debate as to which cells are best to analyze. A small number of centers biopsy the two polar bodies.[15] The first is made at the time of ovulation, the second at the time of fertilization. These cells do not become part of the fetus and are therefore considered somewhat safer to remove. The fact that they include only the maternal contribution to the embryo limits the evaluation.

Most commonly, an embryo is biopsied on the third day from fertilization. It is typically six to eight cells at this time, and one cell (or rarely two) is removed for analysis. There is debate as to whether or not this is harmful to the embryo. Some centers report lower pregnancy rates with PGD than without.[16] The benefits (e.g., disease prevention), however, may outweigh this risk. If there is a risk from the performance of PGD, it is that the pregnancy is less likely to implant successfully. Pregnancies that have progressed to term after performance of PGD have not shown an increased rate of anomalies or birth defects. A limitation of this technique is that the cell biopsied may have a different genetic composition than the rest of the embryo. This phenomenon, which is known as *mosaicism*, can lead to normal embryos being discarded as abnormal and abnormal embryos labeled as normal.

The analysis of the cell(s) usually takes over 24 hours. Meanwhile, the embryo (hopefully) continues to grow. On the fifth day from fertilization the collection of cells has developed different layers and is known as a *blastocyst*. The blastocyst(s) is then transferred into the uterus with a thin catheter. If extra healthy embryos are created they may be frozen for possible future use.[17]

More recently, some centers have biopsied *trophectoderm* cells, cells from the outer layer of a blastocyst. This procedure has two distinct advantages and one significant drawback. The cells obtained are from the future placenta or membranes, not the fetus itself. It also allows the evaluation of several cells from each embryo, thereby decreasing the chance of error based on a single cell. However, because the embryo is already a blastocyst and cannot be maintained in a culture medium for another day or two, this requires freezing the embryos until the diagnosis is known.

In general, IVF centers prefer to transfer fresh embryos because of their higher pregnancy rates compared to embryos frozen and thawed. However, recent advances in freezing techniques, such as vitrification, have resulted in pregnancy rates fairly close to those of fresh embryos. Freezing of embryos in the past was usually performed with what is known as the "slow freeze" technique. Special solutions are used to withdraw water from the embryo, and the cell is cooled at a very controlled rate to decrease the risk of ice crystals forming. Ice crystal formation during the freezing process can severely damage and kill the embryo. The newer technique, vitrification, also uses special solutions, but the embryo is plunged directly into liquid nitrogen, thereby instantaneously causing it to "turn to stone." This technique appears to be superior in freezing embryos at the blastocyst stage.[18]

Array Comparative Genome Hybridization (CGH)

The FISH technique has a significant limitation in that it can look only for a certain number of mutations at a time. Another technique, known as *comparative genome hybridization* (CGH), overcomes this limitation. It uses PCR to enhance the signal of all the chromosomes. The entire genome is amplified, and variations in *single nucleotide polymorphisms* (SNPs) or *copy number variants* (CNVs) are counted by a computer. The computer can further analyze the thousands of individual data points obtained to give information on all the chromosomes, not just those for which a probe is available.

Because of the speed at which this analysis can be performed, a single cell from a day 3 embryo can be successfully analyzed in time to perform transfer prior to five days in the same cycle without the need for freezing.[19] A recent report showed that CGH could even be performed in only several hours, allowing biopsy of several blastocyst cells combined with a fresh embryo transfer the same day.[20] The future of PGD likely resides in this technology, allowing the analysis of many individual genes as well as all the chromosomes quickly and simultaneously.

Donated Gametes

In cases where the genetic mutation cannot yet be tested for, donated gametes are sometimes used, thereby obviating the need for PGD. When eggs are donated from a woman without the genetic condition, IVF must be performed. The IVF techniques described above are then performed on the egg donor instead of the spouse with the genetic condition. When sperm is donated from a man without the genetic disorder, usually only an insemination is needed, not IVF.

Donated gametes raise additional halachic concerns. Egg donation raises questions of who is the halachic mother and from whom it is best to obtain the donation (related vs. unrelated, Jewish vs. non-Jewish).[21] Despite such questions, the procedure has received halachic permission in individual cases of infertility. Donor sperm raises very serious halachic concerns. The obligation to be fruitful and multiply is incumbent on the husband, and use of donor sperm does not fulfill his obligation. Some authorities even feel that this technique is the equivalent of adultery and that the resulting child would be a *mamzer* (the product of a forbidden relationship), with its disastrous ramifications. Others do not agree but nevertheless feel that the procedure should not be done. As always, individual circumstances are taken into consideration. IVF with PGD is halachically preferable to the use of donor gametes. As the mutations underlying the disease are known for more and more conditions, it becomes more and more possible to use the preferable technique.

---

1. Matthew Cohen, MD, is Director of Reproductive Endocrinology at Long Island Jewish Medical Center, an assistant professor at New York University, and a member of the Division of Human Reproduction at North Shore University Hospital.
2. A. H. Handyside, E. H. Kontogiani, K. Hardy, and R. M. L. Winston, Pregnancies from biopsied human preimplantation embryos sexed by Y-specific DNA amplification. *Nature* 1990; 344:768–70.
3. Y. Verlinsky, N. Ginsberg, A. Lifchez, J. Valle, J. Moise, and C. M. Strom, Analysis of the first polar body: preconception genetic diagnosis. *Hum Reprod* 1990; 5:826–29.
4. The needlestick may cause slight bleeding afterwards. It should be noted that this is due to *dam makkah* (bleeding from trauma) in the vagina and thus does not make a woman *niddah*.
5. *Even HaEzer* 22:1.
6. Some, however, maintain that children born via IVF do not fulfill the obligation of *pru urevu*. See, for example, E. Y. Waldenburg, Hafrayat mafchena:diyun refui hilchati. *Sefer Assia* 1986 5:84–93.
7. *Even HaEzer* 23:2.
8. J. L. Simpson, Preimplantation genetic diagnosis at 20 years. *Prenat Diagn* 2010; 30:682–95.
9. See section on The Ethics of Genetic Testing.
10. See section on Genetic Predispositions.
11. T. Hassold, N. Chen, J. Funkhouser, et al., A Cytogenetic Study of 1000 Spontaneous Abortions. *Ann Hum Genet.* London 1980; 44:151–78.
12. D. Warburton, Z. Stein, J. Kline, and M. Susser, Chromosome Abnormalities in Spontaneous Abortion: Data from the New York City Study. In *Human Embryonic and Fetal Death*. L. H. Porter and E. B. Hook (Eds.). New York Academic Press 1980, pp. 261–67.

13. For discussion of gender selection for nonmedical reasons, see the section on Gender Selection.

14. Shaare Zedek hospital, for example, has a committee to approve all such procedures. In general, they will screen only for significant autosomic recessive conditions. In one case to date, however, they did allow it for a woman who was a carrier of a BRCA gene and had already had a number of family members affected by cancer. (Rav Avraham Steinberg, personal communication)

15. The process of producing a female gamete results in the production of one ovum (egg) and three entities that have nuclear material but little cytoplasm. These entities are known as *polar bodies.*

16. S. Mastenbroek, M. Twisk, J. van Echten-Arends, et al., In vitro fertilization with preimplantation genetic screening. *N Engl J Med* 2007, 357:9–17.

17. When the couple does not desire any further children, from a halachic point of view they can be destroyed. See Eliyahu M. Hashmadat, *Beiziot vdilul Ubarim. Techumin* 14:272.

18. W. B. Schoolcraft, E. Fragouli, J. Stevens, S. Munne, M. G. Katz-Jaffe, and D. Wells. Clinical application of comprehensive chromosomal screening at the blastocyst stage. *Fertil Steril*, November 23, 2009 [Epub ahead of print].

19. A. H. Handyside, G. I. Harton, B. Mariani, et al., Karyomapping: a universal method for genome wide analysis of genetic disease based on mapping crossovers between parental haplotypes. *J Med Genet*, October 25, 2009 [Epub ahead of print].

20. R. T. Scott, X. Tao, D. Taylor, K. M. Ferry, and N. R. Treff. A prospective randomized controlled trial demonstrating significantly increased clinical pregnancy rates following 24 chromosome aneuploidy screening: biopsy and analysis on day 5 with fresh transfer. *Fertil Steril* 2010; 94:S2.

21. For further reading see J. D. Bleich, *Contemporary Halachic Problems* Vol IV. New York: Ktav Publishing House, 1995, pp. 237–72; N. Goldberg, *Yichus Imahot b'Hashtalat Ubar b'Rechem shel Acheret. Techumin* 5, pp. 248–59.

Gender Selection

Gender is generally determined genetically by the X and Y or sex chromosomes.[1] In humans, males have one X chromosome and one Y chromosome. Females have two X chromosomes. This difference can be used to select embryos by gender long before one can visually ascertain the gender of the fetus.

It is technically possible to select for gender at three different stages.[2] The first is preconception, before the union of the sperm and the egg. The second is postconception, after the union but before implantation of the embryo into the uterus. The third is after conception, by preventing the birth of the undesired gender.[3]

At the preconception stage, there are a number of techniques. Several methods rely on the timing of marital relations. According to the *Shettles method*, because sperm carrying a Y chromosome are lighter, they swim faster. Therefore, in order to increase the chances of having a boy, one should have relations just prior to ovulation. For a girl, one should have relations three days prior to ovulation. The *O plus twelve* method, on the other hand, claims that for a girl one should have relations 12 hours after ovulation. One problem with these methods is that, other than in articles written by Dr. Landrum Shettles, they have essentially been proven not to work.[4] The other problem, from a Jewish perspective, is the technical difficulty of performing them within the confines of *hilchot niddah*, the laws surrounding the timing of marital relations.[5]

Modified forms of a number of techniques for sperm preparation for *intrauterine insemination* (IUI) have been proposed for gender selection. They all propose separation between X-bearing sperm and Y-bearing sperm, followed by insemination with a portion of the semen meant to be rich in the type of sperm that would lead to the desired gender. A number of techniques have been proposed. The one most commonly used today is the *Ericsson albumin method*. This method, proposed by Dr. Ronald Ericsson, is based on the assumption that Y chromosome-bearing sperm swim faster than X-bearing sperm. Sperm are placed in a test tube on top of a column of layers of albumin and allowed to swim down the column. In the density gradient, or *Percoll method*, the sperm are fractionated by centrifugation through varying layers of density, with the assumption that the heavier X-bearing sperm will sink to the bottom and the lighter Y-bearing sperm will rise to the top. A related method is separation in a *Sephadex column.* In the swim-up method, the sperm are placed under a layer of culture medium and allowed to swim up. In most methods, if the desired gender is a girl, the mother also takes clomiphene citrate. While isolated studies (many co-authored by the proponents of these methods) have shown slightly increased odds for the desired gender, repeated research has found that the processed sperm still has a 50/50 X to Y ratio.

The issue of efficacy is a halachic matter. Jewish law includes much discussion of business ethics. Making a false claim regarding a product is clearly prohibited in the *Shulchan Aruch, Choshen Mishpat* 222. Furthermore, overcharging for a product falls under the prohibition of one's taking advantage of another. One could argue that charging $1,200 for a product that does not work, at least in the sperm separation methods, is forbidden for this reason.

One method of preconception intervention has been shown to be effective in cattle. It is based on *flow cytometry*, a laboratory technique that selects cells according to flow rate. This technique for sperm sorting is based on the fact that the X-bearing sperm are heavier than Y-bearing sperm. Use of this method in humans, known as *Microsort* for the company that performs it, has been shown to be somewhat effective, with 76 percent of the babies born after sorting for Y being male, and 91 percent of the babies born after sorting for X being female.

However, even if the method is shown to be effective, this approach presents halachic difficulties. Production of a sperm sample raises the halachic issue of *hotza'at zera levatala*—the purposeful expulsion of sperm into anything other than the vaginal canal. The *Shulchan Aruch* rules that this is a very serious transgression.[6] Furthermore, in general medical practice, these samples are obtained by self-stimulation. This practice is frowned upon by *halacha*; in the Talmud in *Niddah* 13b it is considered analogous to adultery. The prohibition against self-stimulation is codified as *halacha* in Maimonides' *Mishneh Torah*.[7] These issues have been dealt with extensively in the halachic literature when the procurement is needed to diagnose or treat infertility.[8] It is important to note that while most *poskim* will ultimately permit semen procurement to alleviate the significant suffering that accompanies infertility, it is approved only after considerable grappling with the serious prohibitions. It is not clear that gender selection alone would warrant these leniencies, especially in technologies that have limited success.

Postimplantation gender selection essentially means abortion. This is currently the most common form of gender selection worldwide. Although technically illegal, it has been documented both in India, where providing girls with a dowry is expensive, and in China, which has a one child per family policy; pregnant women undergo ultrasounds for gender determination and then abort females. Abortion is difficult to permit under Torah law, even in the face of significant genetic conditions.[9] Therefore, it is clear that abortion for the purpose of gender selection is not permitted under Jewish law.

The remaining technique is known as *preimplantation genetic diagnosis*, or PGD. To perform PGD, one needs access to the embryo before implantation. Therefore, the embryo is conceived via *in vitro fertilization* (IVF), a process of obtaining sperm from the husband[10] and harvesting the wife's ovum. Harvesting is done under sedation to prevent inadvert moving and usually after the wife has been given medication to cause superovulation so she will produce more eggs for harvesting. The gametes are allowed to join in the laboratory, producing embryos that can be tested.[11]

Regardless of the method of obtaining the genetic material, the amount obtained is miniscule, and special techniques are required to identify the X or Y chromosome. For the purposes of gender selection, this is done by *fluorescent in-situ hybridization* (FISH). A genetic probe is developed that will match a section on the X or Y chromosome. The probe, which has the ability to fluoresce, is put into solution with the genetic material taken from the embryo, and it then matches up with the genetic material. After processing, if a match is found, the genetic material will light up. For example, if a probe is used for the Y chromosome and the sample lights up, the fetus is probably a boy.[12]

The use of medical intervention for gender selection has sparked extensive discussion in general medical ethics. Arguments against allowing the procedure include the fact that it can lead to gender imbalance. The experience of India[13] and China is often brought to support this claim. There are those who feel that use of such medical intervention encourages gender discrimination by making gender important. Many are concerned about the slippery slope to other forms of eugenics. There is mention of the risks of the procedure and its financial costs. On the other hand, those in favor of allowing such intervention point out that many studies have shown that in Western countries people do not prefer boys and parents actually using this technology tend to be evenly split regarding the desired gender.[14] They believe that legislation can prevent slipping down the slippery slope. They argue that the emphasis on risks is overstated and inconsistent, since there is little discussion about the ethics of risks to egg donors who also go through the superovulation procedure, and we allow taking risks for cosmetic surgery. Cost should not be a concern because people pay privately and, first and foremost, people should have the right to choose.

The ambivalence about this technology can be seen in the position statements of major medical organizations. In 1999 the American Society of Reproductive Medicine (ASRM) ruled that the social risks of IVF followed by PGD for gender determination outweigh social benefits and therefore the procedure should be discouraged.[15] The reasons given were that its use could lead to:

- Identification of gender as a reason to value one person over another.
- Gender stereotyping.
- Misallocation of limited medical resources.

It was felt that it was improper to use the technology of IVF for this purpose.

In 2001 the same body ruled that preconception gender selection for nonmedical reasons is an ethically appropriate medical procedure if:

- The method is safe and effective.
- Parents are fully informed of risk of failure.
- Parents affirm that they will accept a child of either sex.
- Parents are counseled regarding unrealistic behavior expectations for a child of the desired gender.
- Parents are offered the opportunity to participate in research regarding the outcomes of gender selection.[16]

The institutional review board of the Center for Human Reproduction took exception to this statement,[17] stating that it is unethical to offer access to sperm sorting but not to PGD, especially because the preconception method is less effective.

The chairman of the ASRM ethics committee responded by stating that programs might ethically offer preimplantation genetic diagnosis for the purpose of gender variety under certain circumstances. This includes having good reason to think that the couple is fully informed of the risks of the procedure and that the couple is counseled against unrealistic expectations regarding the behavior of children of the preferred gender.

The response of the chairman raised quite a furor and a follow-up letter was published,[18] stating that "the need for gender variety in a family does not at this time justify the use of IVF and PGD solely for that purpose" and that IVF and PGD to determine the gender of the first child should be discouraged. It is of interest that the main concern expressed in this letter is that IVF involves the creation and potential destruction of embryos and it is not clear that gender balancing is enough to override this concern. This remains the official position of ASRM to date,[19] despite the fact that in practice, the service is offered in a number of clinics.[20]

The follow-up letter did not quell the debate, as a number of ethicists continue to question why such procedures should be prohibited.[21] However, as it currently stands, both the American Society of Reproductive Medicine and the American College of Obstetricians and Gynecologists[22] rule against PGD being used for gender selection except in the case of sex-linked diseases. In the United States these rulings are recommendations only, so in practice the procedure is done. In much of Europe, however, the practice is outlawed.

So what is the traditional Jewish view on this question?[23] It appears that performing actions meant to produce offspring of a specific gender is not a problem. The Talmud[24] relates how Leah prayed for her male fetus (the future Yosef) to be turned into a female (the future Deena) so Rachel would have at least as many sons as Yaakov's handmaidens. This story is brought by Rashi in praise of Leah, not denigration. The Talmud gives a number of suggestions of how to affect gender.[25] However, note that all these sources prescribe permitted activities, and in fact, mostly laudable activities, such as *havdalah*, charity, prayer, and proper conduct during marital relations. When the needed intervention clashes with other halachic concerns, it is not so simple.

We have already discussed the halachic concerns with the sperm procurement that is needed for both preconception and preimplantation. We will now address the risks of the IVF procedure used in preimplantation gender determination.

One is the risk to the woman undergoing the procedure. In a study of pregnancies in Sweden, women who underwent IVF had an increased risk of ovarian torsion during pregnancy. They were more likely to encounter preeclampsia (63 percent increased risk), placental abruption (over twice the risk), and placenta previa (over three times the risk), all of which pose a significant health risk to the mother.[26] There was an increased use of interventions such as caesarean sections (38 percent increase) and induction of labor (37 percent increase), which have their own attendant risks.[27]

There are also risks for infants born via IVF. Pregnancies achieved by assisted reproduction are at higher risk than spontaneous pregnancies for adverse perinatal outcomes, including perinatal mortality, preterm delivery, and low birth weight. While some of this is related to the increased risk of multifetal pregnancy, singleton pregnancies achieved by assisted reproduction are also at higher risk than spontaneous pregnancies for these problems.[28, 29]

Taking risks with one's health is a halachic issue.[30] The Torah states in *Devarim* 22:8: "If you build a new house you shall make a fence for the roof, and do not cause blood in your house if someone should fall from it." This verse is understood in *halacha* to require the avoidance of harm, as stated in the *Shulchan Aruch Choshen Mishpat* 427:8:

And similarly, anything that presents a danger to life, it is a positive commandment to remove it and to be careful of it and be very cautious in this matter... if he did not remove but rather left these pitfalls that lead to danger he has not fulfilled a positive commandment and has transgressed a negative commandment.

An additional commandment that is linked to the obligation to preserve health is the commandment not to destroy trees (*Devarim* 20:19, *bal tashchit*). This idea is expanded in the commentary of Rav Yechiel Michel Epstein.[31] Additional verses quoted to support the need for preservation of health are *Devarim* 4:9 and *Devarim* 4:15.

Competing *mitzvot* allow for a certain degree of risk. One is allowed to take risks to make a living, as seen in the Talmud's discussion of climbing a ladder as part of one's occupation.[32] Therefore, the concerns of the risks of IVF are generally overridden by the desire to allow the husband to fulfill the commandment of procreation.[33]

Part of the reason for allowing one to enter into IVF despite the numerous halachic issues raised is to alleviate the pain and suffering from lack of children. When the reason for gender selection is to prevent a sex-linked genetic disease, it is clear that the biblical mandate for the physician to heal and the desire to prevent the suffering of the couple from an ill child would override the consideration of danger, and the procedure would be permitted. Similarly, when IVF is being done for other reasons, such as infertility or preventing a genetic disease, and thus there is no added risk, there seems to be no reason to prohibit PGD for gender selection. However, when PGD is done solely for the purpose of family balancing, it is more difficult to permit the risks. Therefore, some halachic authorities, such as Rabbi Yigal B. Shafran, Rabbi Yitzchak Zilberstein, and Rabbi David Bleich, have ruled clearly against PGD for gender selection.[34]

Some have claimed that Judaism has an additional push for gender balance in order to fulfill the commandment to be fruitful and multiply (*pru urevu*). However, a more careful study of this commandment would indicate that this is not the case. The commandment is not fulfilled just by having a boy and a girl, but rather by raising them to the point that they themselves have children.[35] Therefore it is clear that fulfillment of the commandment is something to strive for, but its success is not totally up to us. Furthermore, the Talmud in *Shabbat* 31a relates that at the end of one's life one is asked if one has engaged in *pru urevu*,[36] not if one has reached its ideal fulfillment. To require ongoing attempts at having a child spontaneously is one thing; assuming a need for extraordinary measures is another. Furthermore, fulfilling the mitzvah of *pru urevu* is one of the considerations in halachically permitting contraception, but it is not the only one. Therefore, one should not assume that a woman needs to continue childbearing to the point where it endangers her well-being just because she has children only of one gender.

There will, however, be cases where some halachic authorities feel that the need is great enough to justify performance of PGD. For example, Rabbi Ovadia Yosef permitted PGD for a couple with six children of one sex who were not willing to have more children unless they could be assured that the seventh would be of the opposite gender.[37] Rabbi Mordechai Eliyahu is reported to have permitted gender selection when there are already five children of one gender.[38]

Machon Puah[39] sent a questionnaire on gender selection to a number of prominent rabbis[40] asking whether they would permit a special diet, gender selection of gametes, and/or IVF and PGD. Not surprisingly, in keeping with the idea that wishing for a particular gender is not itself a problem, none of these rabbis had difficulty with the idea of changing the diet. Rabbi Avigdor Nebenzahl felt that sorting would be better than IVF/ PGD, an answer that seemed to indicate that IVF/PGD might be permitted in some situations. Rabbi Shlomo Amar, the Sephardi Chief Rabbi of Israel, felt that those methods that required medical intervention were quite problematic, although they might be allowed in certain extraordinary circumstances. Rabbi Yehoshua Neuwirth expressed his displeasure with the entire topic.

Jewish law has contributed some unique situations where halachic concerns have been sufficient to allow gender selection. One such case involved the wife of a *kohen* whose husband was infertile and who was having a child by IVF. Donor sperm was being used,[41] and therefore the child was not going to have the halachic status of a *kohen*. The couple was concerned that if the child was a boy everyone would thus know that he was conceived in this unusual manner and therefore they desired a girl. This request was approved by the Department of Health, although it engendered a number of questions.[42] Similarly, requests have been approved to have a boy to avoid the problems of a father's being alone with a girl who is not his biological daughter.[43]

As has been mentioned, a recurrent objection to PGD for gender selection in general medical ethics is that it may be the first step down a slippery slope. In other words, it is not the procedure itself that is the problem but where it may lead. In a recent article,[44] Rabbi Yuval Sherlow undertakes an in-depth analysis of the slippery slope contention using PGD for gender selection as his example. He refers to the chance of the slide down the slope actually happening; the seriousness of the consequences of such a slide; and the risk of not allowing a procedure that is in itself innocuous because of fears of the slide. He applies halachic principles such as "One does not make a decree that the majority of the community cannot uphold" (*Ein gozrim gezerah ele im ken rov hatzibur yachol laamod bo*); "The Rabbis did not make decrees on events that were uncommon (*bedavar she-eino matzui lo gazru rabanan*); and "serious loss" (*hefsed merubeh*) to help analyze these issues.

In summary, the jury is still out on the general ethics of this procedure. The Jewish view is not to encourage the procedure, although it might be permitted in certain extraordinary circumstances.

---

1. However, the external appearance can occasionally differ from the genetic makeup, as is discussed in the chapter "Disorders of Sexual Development."

2. There is actually a fourth possibility of gender selection after birth, through infanticide. However, this is so clearly unacceptable both in *halacha* and in Western society that it will not be discussed further. It is of note that this method certainly has been used often throughout human history and goes on today in a number of countries. See for example F. G. Abrejo, B. T. Shaikh, and N. Rizvi,

'And they kill me, only because I am a girl'...a review of sex-selective abortions in South Asia, 2009; 14:10–16.

3. A good lay site for discussion of these methods (but not their halachic aspects) is www.ingender.com. This site includes the references to the scientific journal articles that support and negate each method described here.

4. A. J. Wilcox, C. R. Weinbery, and D. D. Baird. Timing of sexual intercourse in relation to ovulation—effects on the probability of conception, survival of the pregnancy and sex of the baby. *NEJM* 1995; 333:1517–21.

5. Many women ovulate around the time of *mikveh* use. Therefore, a date three days before ovulation is likely to come out before *mikveh* use, when marital relations are prohibited.

6. *Even HaEzer* 22:1.

7. *Hilchot Isurei Biah* 21:18.

8. See, for example, D. R. Zimmerman, *A Lifetime Companion to the Laws of Jewish Family Life*. Jerusalem: Urim Publications, 2005, p. 155.

9. See chapter on Abortion.

10. As was discussed above, the usual methods for sperm procurement are halachically problematic. A specific halachic question should be asked about the permissibility of the procedure and the least problematic methods of obtaining sperm.

11. See chapter on Artificial Reproductive Technology.

12. The reason for the "probably" is that no test in medicine is perfect. Even though, in theory, every cell is genetically similar to every other one, at times division is not perfect. In that case, one can end up with one cell missing something that is present in other cells. Genetic variation among the cells of one individual is known as *mosaicism*.

13. S. M. George, Millions of missing girls: from fetal sexing to high technology sex selection in India. *Prenat Diagn* 2006; 26:604–9.

14. T. Jain, S. A. Missmer, R. S. Gupta, and M. D. Hornstein. Preimplantation sex selection demand and preferences in an infertility population. *Fertil Steril* 2005; 83:649–58.

15. Ethics Committee of the American Society of Reproductive Medicine. Preimplantation genetic diagnosis and sex selection. *Fertil Steril* 1999; 72:595–98.

16. Ethics Committee of the American Society for Reproductive Medicine. Preconception gender selection for nonmedical reasons. *Fertil Steril* 2001; 75:861–64.

17. N. Gleicher, K. Vishvanath. Gender selection for nonmedical indications. *Fertil Steril* 2002; 78:460–462.

18. J. A. Robertson. Sex selection for gender variety by preimplantation genetic diagnosis. *Fertil Steril* 2002; 78:463.

19. Ethics Committee of the American Society for Reproductive Medicine. Preconception gender selection for nonmedical reasons. *Fertil Steril* 2004; 82:S233–3.

20. **ESHRE** PGD **Consortium** Steering Committee. **ESHRE** Preimplantation Genetic Diagnosis **Consortium**: data collection III. *Hum Reprod*, 2002; 17:233–46.

21. B. Steinbock, Sex Selection: Not obviously wrong, Hasting Center Report. Available at www.jstor.org/stable/3528293.

D. Heyd, Male or female, we will create them: the ethics of selection for non-medical reasons. *Ethical Perspectives* 2003; 10:204–14.

22. Sex selection. ACOG Committee Opinion No 360. *Obstet Gynecol* 2007; 109:475–78.

23. Additional discussion of this topic can be found in a topic symposium "Sex selection and halachic ethics; a contemporary discussion," published in *Tradition*, in Spring 2007 (Volume 40, Issue 1, pp. 45–78), and in G. Weizman and D. Harari, Revisiting sex selection in Jewish law. *Conversations* 2010; 1:121–31.

24. *Berachot* 60a.

25. *Berachot* 5b: "R. Chama ben Chanina said in the name of R. Yitzchak—One who orients his bed between north and south will have male children," based on a verse in Psalms 17.

Bava Batra 10b: "What should a person do in order to have male children? R. Eliezer says he should distribute his money to poor people. R. Yehoshua says he should make his wife happy with marital relations."

Shevuot 18b: "R. Chiya bar Abba states in the name of R. Yochanan: One who physically separates from his wife before her expected menses will have sons—based on the juxtaposition of two verses.... R. Chiya bar Abba states in the name of R. Yochanan: One who makes *havdalah* on Saturday night will have male children, based on the same juxtaposition.... R. Binyamin bar Yeffet states in the name of R. Elazar: One who behaves in a holy manner during marital relations will have male children, based on another juxtaposition."

Niddah 31a: "If the woman gives seed first, she has a male, and if the man gives seed first, she will have a female."

26. B. Kallen, O. Finnstrom, K. G. Nygren, P. Otterblad Olausson, and U. B. Wennerholm, In vitro fertilisation in Sweden: obstetric characteristics, maternal morbidity and mortality. *BJOG* 2005 November; 112 (11):1529–35.

27. N. Pallasmaa, U. Ekblad, A. Aitokallio-Tallberg, et al., Cesarean delivery in Finland: maternal complications and obstetric risk factors. *Acta Obstet Gynecol Scand.* 2010 July; 89 (7):896-902.

28. V. M. Allen, R. D. Wilson, and A. Cheung, Pregnancy outcomes after assisted reproductive technology. *J Obstet Gynaecol Can.* 2006 March; 28 (3):220–50.

29. J. P. Aluksl and L. I. Lipshultz, Safety of assisted reproduction, assessed by risk of abnormalities in children born after use of in vitro fertilization techniques.

Nature Clinical Practice. www.nature.com/clinicalpractice doi: 10/1038/ncpuro1045. Accessed July 25, 2010.

30. See, for example, J. David Bleich, *Hazardous Procedures in Judaism and Healing.* New York: Ktav Publishing House, 1981.

31. *Torah Temimah, Devarim* 20:57.

32. *Bava Metzia* 112a.

33. This includes both the commandment of *pru urevu* (be fruitful and multiply, understood as having one boy and one girl—but see source below), which is a Torah-level commandment, and *lashevet* (to keep having children), which is a rabbinic-level commandment.

34. See R. Grazi and J. Wolewolsky, Genetic Screening and Preimplantation Sex Selection in Halacha, *Le'ela* 1993:36. Available at http://www.daat.ac.il/daat/english/ethic/genetic_1.htm. Accessed November 11, 2010.

35. *Shulchan Aruch Even HaEzer* 1:5–6.

36. *Shabbat* 31a.

37. J. B. Wolowelsky and R. V. Grazi, Sex selection and halachic ethics: a contemporary discussion. *Tradition* 2007; 40:45–52. The same issue has articles on that topic from K. Brander, B. Freundel, M. Friedman, J. Goldberg, B. Greenberger, F. Kaplan, E. Reichman, and D. R. Zimmerman, pp. 53–78. Additional reading on this topic can be found in J. A. Klug, A boy or a girl? The ethics of preconception gender selection, *Journal of Halacha and Contemporary Society* 2004; 48:5–27.

38. Ibid.

39. An institute in Israel that assists couples with halachic issues related to infertility. Their website is www.puah.org.il.

40. The original answers can be downloaded at http://www.yutorah.org/_materials/Playing%20G-d1.pdf.

41. Use of donor sperm is itself a halachic controversy.

42. R. V. Grazi and J. B. Wolowelsky, Addressing the idiosyncratic needs of Orthodox Jewish couples requesting sex selection by preimplantation genetic diagnosis (PGD). *J Assist Reprod Genet.* 2006; 23:421–25.

43. Ibid.

44. Y. Sherlow, *Halacha v Hemidron Hachlaklak. Akdamot.*

Abortion

Alan Jotkowitz[1]

Introduction

At this point in history, the prevention of many genetic diseases involves preventing the birth of an affected child. This situation can sometimes be achieved by avoiding marriages between carriers of recessive diseases, or by pre-implantation genetic diagnosis of an infant conceived through in vitro fertilization; however, in many cases neither solution is possible. This leaves the options of abortion or the birth of an affected child.

Abortion is not a simple matter in *halacha*. A *posek* (halachic decisor) who can relate to the circumstances of the couple facing this decision should be consulted. The goal of this chapter is to understand the halachic issues on which individual answers are based.

The Halachic Process

First, it important to realize that *halacha* is case based. The Jewish legal scholar Menachem Elon has described the process as follows:

> In responsa literature the reader is thrust into the midst of a living legal reality, listens to the facts and arguments that the litigants present, and accompanies the decisor (a rabbi who undertakes to issue a halachic ruling) at each stage of his legal inquiry. The problem facing the student and researcher of responsa literature is that [this literature] plunges them into a world of creativity, the inner sanctum of the laboratory. They are partners in experiments, creation, and comprehensive and profound legal analysis. They hear the objective socioeconomic background description that is incorporated into the halachic debate, and they are privy to the explicit or implicit allusions to the decisor's vacillations and efforts to arrive at an answer and a legal solution that both rest on precedent and meet the many needs of his contemporaries.[2]

Therefore, since no two cases can ever be identical, different answers may be given to seemingly similar cases because of subtle differences in individual circumstances.

Sources Used in the Halachic Discussion Regarding Abortion

Inadvertent abortion is mentioned obliquely in the Torah (*Shemot* 21:22–23). It states that if two men are fighting and they strike a pregnant woman and cause her to miscarry, the one who strikes her is obligated to pay the woman's husband for the loss of the fetus.

Abortion is discussed more specifically in the Talmud in *Sanhedrin* 57b. There it states that if a non-Jew performs an abortion, he is guilty of murder. This statement is derived from *Breishit* 9:6, where the Noachide laws (those laws that apply to all descendants of Noach, i.e., all people alive today) are listed. The verse states *hashofech dam ha-adam ba-adam damo yeshafech*. The simple translation is: "One who sheds the blood of a person, by a person shall his blood be shed," meaning that one who spills human blood is liable for capital punishment. However, the prefix *ba-* can mean "in" as well as "by," and by punctuating differently, *dam ha-adam ba-adam* can mean "the blood of a person in (within) a person"—and thus can refer to a fetus. This interpretation would indicate that capital punishment is meted out for the killing of a fetus.

Killing of a fetus by a Jew is discussed in the Mishna in *Oholot* 7:6, which states, "When a woman is having difficulty giving birth, one may dismember the fetus in the womb and remove it limb by limb, because her life takes precedence over his; if most (of the body)[3] has emerged, one may not touch it because one does not put aside one life for another." We can infer from this *mishna* that abortion is permissible in order to save the life of the mother.

The Talmud in *Arachin* 7a states:

Mishna: A [pregnant] woman who is going out to be executed—we do not wait until she gives birth [to execute her]. A woman who is sitting on the birthstool—we wait until she gives birth [before executing her] ….

Gemara: It might seem obvious [that we do not wait for a woman to give birth before executing her], for [the fetus] is part of her body. In fact, it is necessary [to teach this], for you might have thought that since it is written (*Shemot* 21:22) "as the husband of the woman shall cause to be assessed against him," we infer that [the fetus] is the property of the husband, therefore we may not cause him to lose [his property]. The Mishna therefore informs us that we do not wait. But that is indeed so [we should delay the execution to prevent loss to the husband]! Rabbi Abahu said in the name of Rabbi Yochanan, the verse states (*Devarim* 22:22) "and also both of them shall die." [The superfluous word "also"] comes to include the fetus. ....(Regarding) a woman who is sitting on the birthstool, what is the reason [that we wait for the child to be born]? Since the fetus has shifted position [in preparation for birth], it is considered a different body.

The implication of this passage is that before a woman is in labor, the fetus is considered merely the property of the husband and not a separate entity.

Halachic Discussion of Abortion

The key halachic decisors on abortion in modern times are Rabbi Moshe Feinstein and Rabbi Eliezer Waldenberg. Before entering the specifics of the abortion debate, it is important for us to understand their different approaches to halachic rulings.

Rabbi Feinstein writes:

Has the Torah already reached its end and limit, God forbid, that we may rule only regarding what we find in the books—and when new questions arise that are not in the books, we may not decide them even if we have the ability to do so? In my opinion, it is certainly forbidden to say this, for the Torah must continue to become greater, even now in our time. And one who is able to decide questions that come before him—after exploring and analyzing the Talmud and previous decisors with clear understanding and solid proofs, even in a new matter that the books did not address— is obligated to do so.[4]

Regarding rabbinic precedent, he comments:

And even regarding a law that is found in the books, the decisor must certainly understand it and reach his own conclusion before he adjudicates. He should not just adjudicate on the basis of what is in the books, because this is like adjudicating based on superficial understanding.... And even if his decision is against some great *Acharon* [modern sage], what of it? We are certainly allowed to disagree with the *Achronim* and sometimes even with the *Rishonim* [medieval sages] when there are convincing proofs.[5]

This quotation summarizes Rabbi Feinstein's halachic decision-making methodology and gives a glimpse into his remarkable intellectual independence. He also challenges his readers:

I decided to print my responsa because my purpose is only to clarify the *halacha*, and every scholar and decisor should analyze my words and decide for himself whether to rule thus. And you will see that I did not rely like a blind person in a chimney on the prior works of our Rabbis but I checked with all my strength to see if they are correct ...so therefore I request that whoever reads my books should check for himself and then issue a practical ruling.[6]

In contrast, like many of his contemporaries, Rabbi Waldenberg relies much more on the works of previous decisors and quotes extensively from them in his responsa.

Regarding abortion, R. Feinstein maintains that abortion is a form of murder for a Jew or non-Jew; the only difference is that a Jew does not receive capital punishment for performing an abortion.[7] He bases this position on Maimonides'[8] codification of the principle from *Sanhedrin* 57b as follows: "a non-Jew who kills a person, even a fetus in its mother's womb, is sentenced to death" (*Hilchot Melachim* 9:4). Surprisingly, there is no parallel explicit discussion in the Talmud, Maimonides, or the Codes regarding what happens if a Jew aborts a fetus. However, on the basis of the principle that "there is nothing prohibited to a non-Jew that is permitted to a Jew," R. Feinstein reaches his conclusion.

Rav Waldenberg, on the other hand, uses as his primary source the verse from *Shemot* as interpreted by the *Mechilta* (halachic midrash). The perpetrator only has to pay financial compensation to the husband for the value of the fetus but does not receive any additional punishment for the death of the fetus.[9] R. Waldenberg infers from this that the fetus is not considered an independent person, just a monetary asset of the husband.[10]

The significance of the *mishna* in *Oholot* is also debated by Rabbis Waldenberg and Feinstein. Rashi comments on this *mishna*, which allows dismembering of the fetus to save the life of the mother, "as long as the fetus has not emerged, he is not a *nefesh* (person) and one may kill him to save his mother, but when his head has emerged, one may not touch him to kill him, because it is as if he has been born, and one does not put aside one *nefesh* for another."[11] R. Waldenberg feels it is clear from Rashi that before birth the fetus is not considered a person, and that is why abortion by a Jew is not considered murder.[12]

Rabbi Feinstein focuses more on Maimonides' codification of this law, which has engendered great controversy and debate among later authorities. He writes:

A pregnant woman who is having difficulty giving birth, one may dismember the fetus in the womb with a medication or by hand because he is like a *rodef* [the halachic term for a person trying to kill another person] trying to kill her, but if the head has emerged one does not touch him because one does not put aside one life for another, and this is the way of the world.[123]

Maimonides does not offer Rashi's explanation for why one is allowed to kill the fetus in the womb—that the fetus is not considered a person—but suggests that the reason is based on the principle of *rodef*. However, there are three main difficulties with how Maimonides codified this law:

1. Does Maimonides maintain that one is allowed to abort the fetus in the first case only because he considers the fetus a *rodef*, but otherwise it would be murder? Or does he think that abortion is not murder and the introduction of the principle of *rodef* is for another reason, not necessarily to overcome the prohibition of murder?

2. The Talmud in *Sanhedrin* 72b posits that the law of *rodef* does not apply to a fetus whose head has emerged, because the mother is "pursued from Heaven"—her danger in childbirth is considered an "act of God" and not the result of any action on the part of the fetus. So how can Maimonides apply the law of *rodef* to a fetus inside the womb? Shouldn't the exception of being "pursued from Heaven" apply here as well?

3. There also apparently exists an internal conflict in the ruling of Maimonides itself. If the fetus is considered a *rodef* inside the womb, why isn't it also considered a *rodef* when it is partially born? Alternatively, why doesn't Maimonides' explanation of "it is the way of the world" also apply to a fetus in the womb?

Rabbis Feinstein and Waldenberg disagree on the interpretation of the enigmatic text. How they respectively resolve the contradictions directly affects the question of whether a fetus is considered a person. R. Feinstein forcefully maintains that the only reason one is allowed to abort the fetus is based on the principle of *rodef* because Maimonides considers the fetus a person.[14] R. Waldenberg responds to this interpretation of Maimonides,

"I am astounded and perplexed how he [R. Feinstein] ignored or didn't pay attention to the great decisors of previous generations, some of whom even lived close to the time of the *Rishonim*, who explained differently and the opposite," and he maintained that even according to Maimonides a fetus is not considered a person.[15]

The position of Nachmanides[16] also engenders debate between R. Feinstein and R. Waldenberg. Nachmanides, commenting on the *mishna* in *Niddah* 43b–44a, which states that one is sentenced to death for killing a one-day-old infant, asserts:

> But this law does not apply to a fetus because it is not called a person (*nefesh adam*). This is also stated in *Sanhedrin* 72b: A woman who is having difficulty giving birth, we bring a knife and dismember the fetus limb by limb; if the head has emerged we do not touch it because one does not put aside one life for another. We see that [before the head has emerged] there is no issue of saving a life [of the fetus], and the Torah also teaches us that [one who causes a miscarriage only] pays the value of the fetus [to the husband].[17]

It seems clear from the comments of Nachmanides that he feels that a fetus is not considered a person but is a monetary asset of the husband, and therefore one is not liable for abortion. R. Waldenberg deduces from these statements of Nachmanides that, since he does not consider the fetus a person, there is no capital liability for causing the death of a fetus.[18]

The discussion of abortion found in *Arachin*, which implies that the fetus is not a separate entity, presents a challenge to Rabbi Feinstein's thesis, and he takes great pains to explain the passage differently. He claims that the verse from *Devarim* teaches us that it is permitted to kill the fetus even though it is an independent person.[19]

This is a difficult assertion to make for two reasons: First, the Talmud itself seems to imply that the fetus is not a separate person by calling the mother and fetus "one body." Second, the Talmud states that it is obvious that one may abort the fetus before the mother is in labor, and the verse in *Devarim* merely teaches that one may do this even at a financial loss to the husband.

As Lord Rabbi Immanuel Jakobovits and others have pointed out, there is a gap of hundreds of years during which abortion is scarcely mentioned in the halachic literature,[20] and we do not encounter the issue again until the end of the 16th century in the responsa of the Maharit.[21] Even though Rabbis Feinstein and Waldenberg may differ in how authoritative and binding they feel these earlier responsa are, from a halachic method-ological perspective they must address the arguments they raise and the conclusions they reach.

The Maharit was asked whether a Jewish doctor may assist a non-Jewish woman to get pregnant or to miscarry, and whether the latter is considered murder. He answers:

I remember that I saw in the responsum of the Rashba (a promi-nent medieval Talmudist) that he testifies that the Ramban helped a non-Jewish woman get pregnant, and to induce a miscarriage is not considered murder because even the fetus of a Jew is not considered a person... and therefore it seems that for the needs of the mother one may induce a Jewish woman to miscarry, because this is for the health of the mother.[22]

This position of the Maharit seemingly contradicts R. Feinstein's con-tention that abortion is a form of murder. However, R. Feinstein claims that this responsum of the Maharit (number 99) is a "forgery written by a mistaken student in his name." He bases this on two reasons:[23]

1. In an earlier responsum (number 97), the Maharit writes, "we see that there is a dispute as to whether the law of saving a life (*pi-kuach nefesh*) applies to a fetus, and in matters of life and death one should be lenient and save them—and all the more so, one should not harm them." The implication of this statement is that the fetus is considered a person and that abortion is forbidden.
2. The actual responsum of the Rashba that the Maharit quotes does not say that the Ramban aborted non-Jewish fetuses, only that he helped non-Jews get pregnant.

R. Waldenberg responds incredulously to these assertions:
What does R. Feinstein do with these words of the Maharit? He takes the easy way out and writes that you should pay no attention to this responsum because it is definitely a forgery from a mis-taken and misleading student who wrote it in his name. I am per-plexed—how can one uproot an entire responsum of the Maharit on the basis of such an imagined assumption? And this would be even if there were no proof against this, but in practice we do have a proof against this [that the responsum is a forgery].[24]

R. Waldenberg then cites a student of the Maharit who quotes the disputed responsum in his name, thus testifying to its veracity. Regarding the apparent contradiction between the two responsa, R. Waldenberg postulates that in reality responsa 97 and 99 are one responsum and the text quoted above that contradicts responsum 99 should be read simply as the preliminary thoughts of the Maharit.[25] He also claims that the Maharit never suggested that the Ramban aborted fetuses, but the correct reading of the disputed quotation ("the Ramban helped a non-Jewish woman get pregnant and to induce a miscarriage is not considered murder") is to view the sentence as two independent clauses. The first half of the citation is from Rashba, and the second clause begins the words of the Maharit.[26] Another distinguished authority, the Rav Paalim, relies on responsum 99 of the Maharit to permit abortion in certain instances.[27]

R. Feinstein takes the Rav Paalim to task for not also quoting responsum 97 of the Maharit, and suggests that this might be because he didn't have firsthand access to the necessary books.[28] R. Waldenberg responds "that Rabbi Feinstein must not have seen the actual text of the responsum …because the Rav Paalim specifically also cites responsum 97."[29]

Practical Guidelines

Even though R. Waldenberg does not consider abortion murder, he considers it a very serious prohibition. He writes,

All Jews are commanded not to act lightly regarding abortion. And great responsibility is placed both on the one who asks regarding abortion, and on the one who answers. Notwithstanding, the fact that prohibiting abortion is a deterrent against immorality, and even the nations of the world have laws prohibiting abortion with severe punishments.[30]

R. Waldenberg does not clearly state why he feels abortion is prohibited. He mentions several possibilities in his many responsa without clearly committing to one.[31, 32, 33]

1. Many authorities view abortion as falling under the rubric of masturbation, or "wasting seed for naught," which implies that it is forbidden to squander potential life.
2. Prohibition of abortion may be an extension of the prohibition of harming or injuring oneself.
3. The prohibition on abortion may be part of a general halachic directive to populate the world.

R. Waldenberg does not specify the actual source of this prohibition. Apparently, he feels that abortion is only a rabbinic prohibition and therefore it is easier for him to permit abortion if there is a great need. He permits abortion when there is any danger to the mother or any medical reason for the procedure; however, he extends this dispensation to other cases as well. He cites Rabbi Yaakov Emden, who permitted abortion in the case of a married woman who had become pregnant through an extramarital relationship, and then adds, "and even when the fetus is legitimate, there is room to permit for a great need until the fetus is ready to be born, even if it is not in order to save the life of the woman but to save her from a pregnancy which is causing her great pain."[34] R. Waldenberg attaches great significance to the dispensation to permit abortion in cases of great pain, and specifically relates it to the case of a fetus with Tay-Sachs:

> Is there case of greater need, pain and suffering that will be caused to the mother in giving birth to this child, where all indications are that he will suffer and surely die within a few years…and add to this the pain and suffering that the child will experience…. And therefore if *halacha* permits abortion for reasons of pain and suffering and great need, then this should be a classic case for allowing it. And it makes no difference whether the suffering is physical or emotional, because in many instances emotional suffering is greater than physical suffering.[35]

For reasons of self-respect, dignity, and avoiding desecration of the name of God, he also permits a married woman to have an abortion if the pregnancy was the result of an affair or a rape. R. Waldenberg also permits a nursing woman to have an abortion because of the fear that she will no longer be able to nurse, which is a potential danger to the nursing infant. This ruling is somewhat surprising, since there are reasonable alternatives to nursing currently available.[36]

It is clear that R. Waldenberg's relatively liberal position on abortion is not based on a woman's right to choose. In other contexts, he has written forcefully that a person does not have the right to decide what will happen to his body, because in reality all life belongs to God. For example, in regard to terminal care, he maintains that the physician is required to do everything in his power to compel the patient to extend his life.[37]

R. Feinstein does not permit abortion in any of these cases of emotional need and even restricts abortion in situations of potential danger to the woman. As he had explained, allowing abortion is based on the principle of *rodef* and not on the general dispensation that one may violate the laws of the Torah to save a life. There are legal differences between these principles. The general dispensation also applies in situations of doubt; in other words, even if one is not sure if there is danger to life, one is allowed to violate the Torah in order to save a life. In order to classify someone as a *rodef*, one must be certain that he intends to murder the victim. Therefore, according to R. Feinstein, it must be highly certain that the pregnancy is life threatening to the woman before an abortion is permitted.[38]

The genetic condition most discussed in modern printed responsa regarding abortion is Tay-Sachs disease. In this case R. Waldenberg is willing to permit even a late-term abortion[39] to prevent the suffering of the parents, and R. Feinstein is not willing to permit even an early abortion. However, what about genetic diseases that are not fatal but lead to mild to moderate impairments such as Down syndrome? Does abortion for a fetus with Down syndrome meet the requirement of "great need" as mandated by Rabbi Waldenberg? This is obviously a much more difficult question because of the uncertain prognosis of children with Down syndrome and the varied ability of families to cope with the affected child. Rabbi Waldenberg himself is hesitant about giving a general dispensation to allow abortion for a fetus with Down syndrome but instead instructs a couple to talk to their personal rabbi, who will be better able to assess their ability to cope with the child. However, he notes there is certainly room to allow an abortion in selected cases because the birth of a child with Down syndrome has the potential "to destroy the psychological well-being of the wife and husband and also put them at risk for a serious or minor illness and also destroy their way of life."[40]

Other genetic conditions have not been addressed in the halachic literature as extensively as Tay-Sachs. However, in issuing rulings to specific couples, the responsa discussed above are used as paradigms. It is easy to understand that a ruling on Canavan disease will be similar to one on Tay-Sachs because the clinical course is similar. If there is hesitation in allowing abortion in cases of a potentially complex disability such as Down syndrome, there is likely to be much more hesitation in cases of single disability such as congenital deafness.

On the basis of a responsum of the Chavat Yair,[41] R. Waldenberg maintains that abortion is more easily permitted earlier in the pregnancy. The Chavat Yair postulates that *halacha* might recognize different legal stages of pregnancy. Before 40 days from conception,[42] the Talmud refers to an embryo as "mere fluid," and at three months the Talmud says that a woman is considered recognizably pregnant. However, none of these talmudic statements relates directly to the legal question of the status of a fetus, and the Chavat Yair himself admits that their relevance to abortion is highly speculative. Nevertheless, many halachic authorities use these stages in their decision making.

R. Waldenberg also recognized these stages but pointed out that the only stage recognized in the Talmud is in *Arachin*, which differentiates before and after the woman sat on the birthstool.[43] Based on this distinction, he permitted abortion of a Tay-Sachs baby up until the end of the seventh month. He brings support for the permissibility of a late-term abortion from the responsum of the Rav Paalim, alluded to above, who was asked whether a woman who was five months pregnant as the result of an adulterous relationship was permitted to have an abortion. He answered,

I do not want to permit or forbid this matter and I will just bring what I found in the responsa of the *Achronim*, who spoke about this....And see the responsum of the Maharit #99, where he says that one can help a Jewish woman miscarry if this is for the mother's needs. And see what he wrote in responsum #97. We see in #99 he permitted abortion because of a maternal need. And it seems to me that there is room to say that where there is a stain on the family, shame, or desecration of the name of God if the fetus is not aborted, that this is considered a great need.

This position of R. Waldenberg was highly controversial and earned him much disdain in the Orthodox world. Rabbi Feinstein had difficulty accepting even abortion within 40 days of conception and suggests that it might be permitted for a non-Jew but not for a Jew.[44]

In conclusion, it is important to note that every situation has its own medical, social, and emotional complexities, which the *posek* has to factor into his decision making. In this vein, Rabbi Aharon Lichtenstein writes:

The question of abortion involves areas in which the halakhic details are not clearly fleshed out in the Talmud and *Rishonim*, and in addition the personal circumstances are often complex and perplexing. In such areas there is room and in my opinion an obligation for a measure of flexibility. A sensitive *posek* recognizes the gravity of the personal situation and the seriousness of the halakhic factors. ...He may reach for a different kind of equilibrium in assessing the views of his predecessors, sometimes allowing far-reaching positions to carry great weight and other times ignoring them completely. He might stretch the halakhic limits of leniency where serious domestic tragedy looms, or hold firm to the strict interpretation of the law, when as he reads the situation, the pressure for leniency stems from frivolous attitudes and reflects a debased moral compass.[45, 46]

1. Dr. Alan Jotkowitz is Professor of Medicine and Director of the Jakobovits Center for Jewish Medical Ethics Ben Gurion University of the Negev and a senior physician at Soroka University Medical Center both in Beersheva Israel.
2. Elon, M. *Ha-mishpat ha-'ivri* (Jewish law). Jerusalem: Magnes, 1973. Part III, p.1215.
3. There are different versions of the text of the *mishna*. In one version it states most of the head. In another it states most of the body.
4. *Iggrot Moshe, Yoreh Deah* 101.
5. Ibid.
6. Preface to *Iggrot Moshe*, Vol. I, and see M. D. Tendler, *Introduction in Responsa of Rav Moshe Feinstein*. New York: Ktav Publishing House, 1996.
7. *Iggrot Moshe, Choshen Mishpat* 2:69.
8. Rabbi Moshe ben Maimon (Rambam); 1125–1204, Spain and Egypt.
9. *Mechilta of Rabbi Shimon ben Yochai*, Chapter 8.
10. *Tzitz Eliezer* 9; 51:3:1:7. The question of whether a fetus is considered a person might be related to another question that the Talmud raises in a number of places. Is a fetus considered in a legal sense an appendage of the mother? See, for example, *Bava Kama* 78b, *Nazir* 51a, and *Gittin* 23b.
11. *Sanhedrin* 72b, Rashi s.v. *yotza rosho.*
12. *Tzitz Eliezer* 9; 51:3:1:3.
13. Rambam, *Mishneh Torah, Hilchot Rotzeach* 1:9.
14. *Iggrot Moshe, Choshen Mishpat* 2:69:1. Rabbi Feinstein himself resolves the difficulties with the Rambam by explaining that when the fetus is partially born, both the fetus and mother are considered *rodfim* because only one of them is able to live. In this situation the Talmud teaches that it is better not to actively sacrifice one life for another. When the fetus is not yet born, only the fetus is considered legally a *rodef.*
15. *Tzitz Eliezer* 14:100:3.
16. Rabbi Moshe ben Nachman (Ramban), 1194–1270; Spain and Israel.
17. *Chidushei HaRamban, Niddah* 44b.
18. *Tzitz Eliezer* 9:51:3:2:5.
19. *Iggrot Moshe, Choshen Mishpat* 2:69:3. In referring to the fetus as an independent entity, the Talmud in *Arachin* uses the Hebrew word *guf*, which

is commonly translated as a body. It is not clear to me if this is different from the terminology Rashi used to refer to the fetus as an independent entity *nefesh*, commonly translated as "person."

20. Immanuel Jakobovitz, *Jewish Medical Ethics*. New York: Bloch Publishing, 1975.

21. Rabbi Yosef Trani, 1568–1639; Israel and Turkey.

22. *Responsa Maharit* Part 1:99.

23. *Iggrot Moshe, Choshen Mishpat* 2:69:3.

24. *Tzitz Eliezer* 14:100:5.

25. Ibid.

26. Among the proofs he brings for the contention that they are one responsum is that in responsum 97 the Maharit writes, "And we see that a fetus is not considered a person and it is permitted for a Jew to abort the fetus of a non-Jew, but one should not do so because of *lifnei iver*, since they are not allowed to have abortions." But logically this citation belongs in responsum 99, where the Maharit is dealing with the question of whether a Jewish physician can perform an abortion on a non-Jew.

27. Rav Paalim, Part 1, *Even HaEzer* #4.

28. *Iggrot Moshe, Choshen Mishpat* 2:69:3.

29. *Tzitz Eliezer* 14:100:5.

30. *Tzitz Eliezer* 9:51:3.

31. Ibid.

32. *Tzitz Eliezer* 14:100:2.

33. *Tzitz Eliezer* 13:102:1.

34. *She'elat Yavetz*, part 1:43. Rabbi Emden himself suggests that one should be more lenient when the pregnancy is the result of an illicit relationship, because in that situation the woman would be liable to the death penalty, and the fetus would be killed along with her. Both Rabbis Feinstein and Waldenberg argue vigorously against this assertion.

35. *Tzitz Eliezer* 13:102:1.

36. *Tzitz Eliezer* 9:51:3.

37. *Tzitz Eliezer* 18:62.

38. *Iggrot Moshe, Choshen Mishpat* 2:69:1.

39. Rabbi Mordechai Willig stated in a lecture in Yeshiva University on April 2, 2008, that since children are viable at an earlier stage today, abortion should be prohibited starting in the fifth month (available at http://www.yutorah.org/lectures/lecture.cfm/723169/Rabbi_Mordechai_I._Willig/Abortion).

40. *Tzitz Eliezer* 14:101:2.

41. Rabbi Yair Chaim Bachrach, 1638–1702; Germany.

42. These 40 days are calculated from the date the woman immersed in the *mikveh* (unless more detailed information on conception is available). This reckoning differs from the medical convention of dating a pregnancy from the beginning of the last menses.

43. *Tzitz Eliezer* 13:102:2.

44. *Iggrot Moshe, Choshen Mishpat* 2:69:1.

45. A. Lichtenstein, Abortion: A halakhic perspective. *Leaves of Faith* Vol. 2. Jersey City, NJ, Ktav Publishing House, 2004. Rabbi Lichtenstein expands on these views in the same book in another article, titled, "The Human and Social Factor in Halakhah."

46. For further reading on the topic of abortion of severely affected fetuses see M.Tzuriel, *Hapalat Ubar Sheuvchana etzlo machala kasha. Techumin.* Available online at www.zomet.org.il/?CategoryID=260&ArticleID=277&print=1.

Consanguineous Marriage

In consanguineous marriages, both partners are descendants of a common ancestor. A large proportion of the world encourages such marriages. It is estimated that 20 percent of the world's population lives in communities with a preference for consanguineous marriage, and that at least 8.5 percent of children worldwide have parents related at the level of second cousins or closer.[1] Advantages cited include preservation of wealth within the family and a presumed better relationship with one's in-laws.

These marriages, however, have been shown to have disadvantages. Many genetic diseases were first discovered in families in which the parents were related. This stands to reason, since the members of a consanguineous couple share more genes than people who are not related. If these shared genes include a mutation that causes an autosomal recessive disease, their children stand a higher chance of getting two defective alleles and thus the disease.[2] First cousins, for example, share one-eighth of their genes. Their children will therefore be homozygous for one in 16 genes.[3]

In the last century, the risk of increased disease in "inbred" families has been stressed. As an outgrowth of this emphasis, cousin marriages are restricted by law in a large number of U.S. states, although they are permitted in the United Kingdom and Australia.[4] Some of these U.S. states will allow the marriage as long as there are no children born of the union. A number of non-Western countries such as China and India have tried to ban cousin or uncle-niece marriages, but with varied success.

Review of the science behind these claims is less clear. As common as the practice is worldwide, the risk of the deleterious outcomes has been difficult to quantify.[5] Many of the countries where such marriages are common also tend to have less developed medical care. Therefore, conditions that could be lethal in those countries may be compatible with a reasonable quality of life in a more developed country. It is also difficult to determine if health problems are caused by consanguinity or by the living conditions in the rural areas where many of these marriages take place.

One of the most accurate studies conducted to date was the Birmingham Birth Study published in 1993. This compared 956 Pakistani babies with 2,432 North European babies all living in Birmingham, England.

The percentage of consanguinity in the Pakistani babies was 69 percent, including 57 percent at the first-cousin level. The percentage in North Europeans was 0.4 percent. The birth prevalence of all congenital and genetic disorders was 4.3 percent in the North Europeans and 7.9 percent in the Pakistanis.[6] The prevalence of conditions that could be linked to recessive inheritance was .28 percent versus 3-3.3 percent.[7]

There are two ways to look at these statistics, both of them correct. One approach is to say that the risk of any defect is twice as great and the risk of a recessive defect is 10–13 times higher when parents are closely related. This approach would indicate that such marriages pose a serious health hazard and significant effort should be put into their prevention. This has been the approach in the past—and it has been shown not to work. For many people who are being "educated," the cultural advantages outweigh the risks.

Another approach is to say that the vast majority (over 90 percent) of children born to related parents are born healthy. In fact, the Genetic Interest Group (GIG), a British national alliance of patient support groups for those affected by genetic disorders,[8] feels the proper approach is to prevent the birth of affected children,[9] not to prevent marriage or pregnancies. Therefore, they recommend the provision of genetic counseling services to communities where the practice is common.

What about the Jewish approach? Biblical sources seem to encourage this practice. Avraham sent his servant to Haran for the specific purpose of finding a related wife for Yitzchak. Yitzchak and Rivka were first cousins once removed. Yaakov was sent there by his parents for this purpose as well. Rachel and Leah were related to Yaakov on both sides. On his mother's side they were first cousins; on his father's side they were second cousins once removed. While the laws of *arayot* (prohibited marriages) prevent the union of parents, siblings, or nephews and aunts, uncle-niece and cousin marriages are permitted.

The Talmud, in fact, contains a dictum encouraging uncle-niece marriages,[10] and this dictum was codified as *halacha* by the Rambam[11] as well as by Rabbi Moshe Isserles (the Rema, Poland,1520–1572) in his gloss on the *Shulchan Aruch*.[12] On the other hand, Rav Yehuda Hachasid counseled against such marriages in his will. A number of halachic authorities have tried to reconcile the contradiction by stating that he was talking only to his family[13] or that times have changed and what may once have been a good idea is no longer appropriate.[14]

The sources above were written before the current medical knowledge regarding the risks involved. Consanguineous marriages were tradition-al in many Jewish communities, especially those from the Middle East. Cousins can spontaneously decide they want to marry even in communi-ties where such marriages are not the norm. Would *halacha* permit this or not? Does the halachic imperative to preserve health[15] prohibit such a practice today?

Such a question was asked of Rav Eliezer Waldenberg by Rabbi Dr. Avraham Steinberg.[16] Rav Waldenberg ruled that we cannot halachically outlaw such marriages, but we can discourage them on the basis of cur-rent knowledge. Rav Ovadia Yosef defended this practice in communities where it was common.[17] A number of articles were published around 1970 in a similar vein of discouraging but not forbidding.[18]

Since the degree of risk can now be better quantified, it seems that these questions should be addressed again. The knowledge that the risk of recessive diseases increases would seem to strengthen the practice of not actively encouraging such unions. On the other hand, should a cousin cou-ple desire to get married, tools are now available to help them. Premarital genetic counseling can help search the family tree for repeated cases of similar pathology that suggests a recessive condition in the family. Link-age analysis within the family can yield association of the condition with genetic markers, for which the couple can then be tested. Recessive condi-tions with known genes that are expected in the ethnic group of the couple can be tested for. Armed with this knowledge, the couple can determine their risk or lack of it. As additional genes are discovered, decisions can be made regarding preconception testing. Such testing can help couples make a more accurate individual halachic decision regarding the proposed union. In the absence of a known condition in the family or positive testing for mutations, the risk a couple is taking would likely fall in the category of halachically acceptable.

Sources

R. I. Bennet, A. G. Motulsky, A. Bittles, et al., Genetic counseling and screening of consanguineous couples and their offspring: recommenda-tions of the National Society of Genetic Counselors. *Journal of Genetic Counseling* 2002; 11:97–119.

Human Genetics Commission, *Cousin Marriages*. Available at www.hgc.gov.uk/client/content.asp?contentID=741

B. Modell and A. Darr, Genetic counseling and customary consanguineous marriage. *Nature Reviews* 2002; 3:225–29.

---

1. B. Modell and A. Darr. Science and society: genetic counseling and customary consanguineous marriage. *Nat Rev Genet* 20023:225–29.
2. They are *not* at a higher risk of inheriting a dominant condition or an X linked disorder. This is somewhat ironic, since a classic story brought to discourage "inbreeding" is the high prevalence of hemophilia in European royal families that has been traced back to Queen Victoria. However, the risk to sons of female carriers is 50 percent and the risk to daughters of affected males is zero, regardless of whether the couple is related or not.
3. This proportion can also be expressed as 0.0625. This percentage is known as the *coefficient of inbreeding*. Calculation of this coefficient helps to quantify the degree of closeness of more complex cases such as marriage of persons who are first cousins on both sides.
4. http://www.cousincouples.com/?page=states
5. A list of published articles on the health risks of consanguinity can be found at www.consang.net.
6. The reasons for the excess of birth defects in addition to those that are known to be genetic can be an ethnic difference in the frequency (separate from consanguinity), environmental factors, or recessive genetic conditions not yet identified.
7. S. Bunday and H. Aslam, A five-year prospective study of the health of children in different ethnic groups with particular reference to the effect of inbreeding. *Eur J Hum Genet* 1993; 206–219.
8. www.gig.org.uk
9. This can be early diagnosis followed by abortion or preimplantation genetic diagnosis and in vitro fertilization. The latter has far fewer halachic problems. See earlier sections on genetic testing, abortion, and artificial reproduction technology for further discussion.
10. *Yevamot* 62b–63a and *Sanhedrin* 76b:
האוהב את שכיניו, והמקרב את קרוביו, והנושא את בת אחותו, והמלוה סלע לעני בשעת דחקו,
עליו הכתוב אומר: (ישעיהו נ"ח) אז תקרא וה' יענה תשוע ויאמר הנני.
11. *Hilchot Isurei Biah* 2:14:
ומצות חכמים שישא אדם בת אחותו והוא הדין לבת אחיו שנאמר ומבשרך לא תתעלם
12. Rema *Even HaEzer* 2:6: ומצוה לאדם שישא בת אחותו וי"א אף בת אחיו
13. *Noda BeYehuda* Tania *Even HaEzer* 79.
14. *Divrei Chaim* Chelek Aleph 8.
15. See section on Gender Selection for discussion of sources.
16. *Tzitz Eliezer* 15:44.

17. *Yabia Omer* 2 *Even HaEzer* 7.
18. Further reading can be found in the articles of *Noam* 12 1969: A. Young 214–26, D. N. Slonim 217–21, Y. Glickman 269–82; and *Noam* 13 1970, *Chatufa Aleph* 83–103.

Section II:
Genetic Diseases

Introduction

With each passing day, genetic causes are found for more and more diseases. At times there is a direct link between the gene and the disease, and sometimes possessing the gene means having a predisposition for an illness. Due to the plethora of genetic diseases, significant thought had to be put into the question of what to include in this book.

It was clear from the onset that "Jewish genetic diseases" would feature prominently. This term refers to diseases that occur more frequently in the Jewish population than the general population, or in which a particular genetic mutation occurs in the Jewish population at a markedly greater frequency. However, deciding which of these diseases to include was difficult. The website of the Israel Department of Health lists 185 Mendelian Disorders found among Jews,[1] far too extensive for a book meant for the general public. Therefore, the list was pared to those conditions with a carrier frequency of approximately 1:100 or more. Conditions that have been found only in isolated families, or only in consanguineous marriages, were omitted. Apologies to those whose particular disease of interest was omitted.

Early on, a decision was made not to focus specifically on conditions that affect the Ashkenazi Jewish population, for two reasons. First, non-Ashkenazim[2] are a large part of the Jewish world. Second, the general focus of most North American articles on Jewish genetic diseases is on the Ashkenazi Jewish community.[3] This emphasis tends to lead to a skewed view of the dangers of being Ashkenazi. Furthermore, with the migrations and redistributions of Jewish communities over the last century and a half, and the *kibbutz galuyot* (ingathering of the exiles) to Israel, the frequency of marriage between people of different ethnic backgrounds has increased.

Then came the question of how to organize the list of diseases. It was tempting to divide them by ethnic origin. However, over time the lines have become blurred. For example, a classic Ashkenazi genetic condition, factor XI deficiency, has also been found among Jews in Iraq. A mutation in the gene associated with familial Mediterranean fever, a classic Sephardi condition, has been found to be quite common among Ashkenazim. Furthermore, with the increased marriage between people of different ethnic backgrounds, the lines between places of origin are becoming blurred.

Another possible method of organization was by the primary organ or system that is affected. However, since many of these conditions affect more than one system, it would not have been clear how to place them. Therefore, it was decided to list the conditions in alphabetical order according to the most common nomenclature for the condition. Alternate names appear throughout the listing with cross-reference to the full description of the condition.

However, discussion of Jewish genetic diseases is not sufficient. While the focus of the book is the Jewish community, and there are diseases that occur more frequently among Jewish populations, Jews also are likely to be affected by diseases for which an ethnic predilection has not (yet?) been found. Therefore, a section on common genetic conditions is included. This section addresses conditions such as Fragile X and spinal muscular atrophy (SMA), as well as chromosomal abnormalities such as trisomy 21 (Down syndrome) and Turner syndrome. These diseases were chosen both because of their frequency and for what they teach us about genetics. Here too the list is not exhaustive. Due to the unique halachic issues involved, a chapter is dedicated to disorders of sexual development, many of which are results of genetic mutations and some of which are discussed in other chapters as well.

The goal of the book is to familiarize the reader with medical conditions that have a genetic basis. It is not meant to be a full medical textbook on these diseases. For this reason, a standard template is provided for each condition. This includes:

- A **summary** and short description of the condition.
- A brief **historical background** of what we know about the condition. This helps put our current genetic knowledge in a historical context and, where relevant, to tell a bit about the person for whom the condition was named.
- A section describing when this condition is suspected and how it is generally **diagnosed**.
- The **genetic cause** section aims to provide as much information as is currently known regarding the linkage between a gene and the condition.
- The **heredity** section includes discussion of the particular mutations that are found in the Jewish community. Carrier frequencies of mutations common in the Jewish community are given. Note that calculations of carrier frequencies are based on testing individuals. Therefore, as the number of individuals

tested and the location of the testing varies, different carrier frequencies may appear in different sources. These numbers should be taken as estimates and not absolute figures.

- Because an entire book could be written on many of the individual conditions discussed, references are provided for additional reading. Those listed as sources are the ones, often professional journal articles, that were used in the compilation of the section. Those listed as further reading are generally writings geared for the general public.

- It is important to realize that genes and descriptions of diseases are not just discussions in print, but conditions that real people live with on a daily basis. It was the author's impression that since many descriptions for the general public are in the context of convincing people to be tested, the descriptions tend to be black and white and quite frightening. The goal in this book is to stress that life goes on. The people who have these conditions continue to live, some with greater struggles and some with less. Therefore a section is provided as to important points regarding **living with the condition**. These are obviously not meant to be a substitute for medical care, but rather an outline of issues involved.

- Last, and certainly not least, **support organizations** exist to help people dealing with the condition live to their fullest potential. A list of these is provided with each condition as well.

---

1. http://www.health.gov.il/Download/pages/bookjews2011.pdf.

2. The term "Sephardi" (literally, "Spanish") is often used to refer to non-Ashkenazi Jews. While this terminology is not completely accurate (many "Sephardi" communities, such as those in Iran and Iraq, did not originate with the exile from Spain, and actually predate the Spanish community), it is common usage in English, and the term "Sephardi" is sometimes used in this book to refer to non-Ashkenazi Jews in general.

3. See, for example, the *Annual Report of Jewish Genetic Diseases* published by Forward.com. Available at http://www.forward.com/articles/11430. The Victor Center for Jewish Genetic Diseases website also provides the Ashkenazi list: http://www.victorcenters.org/Faqs/jewish_genetic.cfm. The lack of discussion of Sephardi conditions has begun to be noted in the United States as well. See, for example, Talia Bloch, "The Other Jewish Genetic Diseases: With Ashkenazic Disorders Getting All the Attention, America's Sephardic Jews Often

Lack Specialized Screening Programs," *Jewish Daily Forward*, August 28, 2009. Available at http://www.forward.com/articles/112426/#ixzz12Ds1wLeI. Accessed October 13, 2010.

Genetic Diseases
with a Jewish Association

Abetalipoproteinemia

Summary

Abetalipoproteinemia is a condition in which fats cannot be absorbed. This leads to very low levels of fats and cholesterol in the blood and inability to gain weight (often called failure to thrive). Fat that is not absorbed is excreted with bowel movements, leading to frothy, smelly stools (*steatorrhea*). The lack of absorption of fat can lead to bloating and abdominal distention. Because a number of vitamins are generally absorbed with fat, people with this condition also suffer from vitamin deficiencies, especially vitamins A and E, and develop the signs of these vitamin deficiencies such as night blindness and neurological degeneration.

Neurological degeneration generally begins at a later age than the gastrointestinal symptoms. The first symptom is usually unsteadiness when walking. This is followed by lack of ability to maintain balance and to stand, generally by the third decade of life. This can be accompanied by muscle weakness. Intellectual development, however, is generally normal.

Visual difficulty also begins at a later age than the gastrointestinal symptoms. The first symptom noted is usually difficulty seeing, particularly at night. The visual difficulties progress because of pigmentary changes in the retina, a condition known as *retinitis pigmentosa*.

The blood cells of people with this condition are malformed. Under the microscope, some of the red blood cells appear star-like (a condition known as *acanthytosis*). Abnormal blood cells are removed from the system at a more rapid rate than normal, and this increased pace of blood cell removal can lead to anemia.

Dietary changes have been shown to help this condition. Restriction of certain fats (triglycerides containing long chain fatty acids) and supplementation of the diet with vitamin E appear to inhibit the progression of the neurological and visual symptoms. The diagnosis is based on the clinical features and the findings of acanthocytes in the blood smear. The diagnosis is supported by the lipid profile that is characteristic for the disease.

A recent study has shown that the genetic mutation in this condition also affects the immune system.[1]

Historical Background

A link between acanthocytosis, atypical retinitis pigmentosa, and *ataxia* (lack of coordination of muscle movements) was reported in 1950 by Dr. Frank A Bassen, a physician, and Dr. Abraham L. Kornzweig, an ophthalmologist, working at Mt. Sinai Hospital in New York. The disease is thus sometimes known as Bassen-Kornzweig syndrome.

Diagnosis of Condition

The condition may be suspected when an infant fails to grow well and has abnormally odorous, copious stools. The suspicion is strengthened when there are abnormal red blood cells on a blood test, worsening loss of balance, and/or worsening vision, especially at night. Blood tests that show extremely low levels of cholesterol and triglycerides are characteristic of this condition. An intestinal biopsy that shows accumulation of lipids in intestinal cells (because people with this condition lack the ability to secrete them) confirms the diagnosis. If a particular mutation is suspected because of family history or ethnic background, molecular genetic testing can be performed.

Genetic Cause

In patients of Ashkenazi Jewish descent, the mutation causing the condition is found within the MTTP gene on the long arm of chromosome 4. This gene codes for a protein involved in the transfer of fat molecules out of intestinal and liver cells.

The most common mutation in this gene is known as G865X.[2]

Heredity

The condition is inherited in an autosomal recessive manner. In order to have the symptoms of the disease, a person must have a mutation on both copies of the gene. Carrier frequency of the G865X mutation in the Ashkenazi Jewish population is 1:113.

Living with the Condition

Treatment is primarily dietary. Fat intake is limited and concentrated on those types of fats that are easier to absorb. Protein is limited as well to about five ounces (140 grams) of lean meat, fish, or poultry. Supplementary vitamins, especially vitamin E, are given. Supervision by an experienced dietician is important.

People with the condition should be followed by an eye doctor to detect early stages of retinal degeneration and to attempt to retain as much vision as possible at each stage. Assistance can be given for learning to deal with the progressive visual disability. Without treatment, most people with this condition will become legally blind. However, early onset of dietary intervention may improve this prognosis.

Dietary management seems to at least delay the neurologic decline. However, should there be neurological difficulties, physical and occupational therapy can be helpful for learning how to cope with the disabilities.

Before the mechanism of this condition was understood, most of those affected died of malnutrition at a young age. With proper dietary management, life expectancy is currently well into adulthood.[3]

Sources
R. Zamel, R. Khan, R. L. Pollex, and R. A. Hegele, Abetalipoproteinemia: two case reports and literature review. *Orphanet Journal of Rare Diseases* 2008, 3:19.
E. Granot and R. Kohen, Oxidative stress in abetalipoproteinemia patients receiving long-term vitamin E and vitamin A supplementation. *Am J Clin Nutr* 2004; 79:226–30.
A. L. Kornzweig, Bassen-Kornzweig Syndrome: Present Status. *Journal of Medical Genetics* 1970; 7:271–76.
J. Zlotogara, Mendelian Disorders Among Jews. http://www.health.gov.il/ Download/pages/bookjews2011.pdf.

Further Reading
Abetalipoproteinemia. Genetics Home Reference.
http://ghr.nlm.nih.gov/condition/abetalipoproteinemia
Abetalipoproteinemia. Madison's Foundation
www.madisonafoundation.org/index2php?option=com_ empower&diseaseID=60

Support Organizations
A Cure for Bassen-Kornzweig Foundation
902 North Richmond, 1st Floor
Chicago, IL 60622
Phone: (773) 486-9247

Email: info@bassenkornzweigfoundation.org
Internet: www.bassenkornzweigfoundation.org
Abetalipoproteinemia Collaboration Foundation
PO Box 8293
Cincinnati, OH 45208
Phone: (513) 557-3808
Email: info@abetalipoproteinemia.org
Internet: www.abetalipoproteinemia.org

Specifically for the retinitis pigmentosa:
RP International
PO Box 900
Woodland Hills, CA 91365
Phone: (818) 992-0500
Fax: (818) 992-3265
Email: info@rpinternational.org
Internet: www.rpinternational.org

Foundation Fighting Blindness
7168 Columbia Gateway Drive, Suite 100
Columbia, MD 21046
Phone: (800) 683-5551
Fax: (410) 363-2393
Internet: www.blindness.org

---

1. S. Zeissig, S. K. Dougan, D. C. Barral, et al., Primary deficiency of microsomal triglyceride transfer protein in human abetalipoproteinemia is associated with loss of CD1 function. *J Clin Invest* 2010; 120: 2889–99.

2. The genetic mutation that is most common in those of Ashkenazi Jewish descent is a switch of glutamine (G) to thiamine (T) in position 2593 of exon 18 of the MTTP gene. This altered code calls for termination of the translation of the microsomal triglyceride transfer protein instead of the glycine amino acid at that point. The MTT protein is thus too short and less functional. The mutation c.2212delT (where T is deleted at position 2212) also occurs in this population, but less frequently.

3. Because this is a rare condition, it is difficult to have enough epidemiologic evidence to give specific figures.

Ataxia-Telangiectasia

Summary

Ataxia-telangiectasia is a condition in which there are progressive neurological symptoms combined with spider-like blood vessels that are apparent in the eyes and skin. The neurological decline generally begins between the ages of one and four years (there is also an adult onset form of the disease). Neurological difficulties include *ataxia* (lack of coordination of muscle movements) that begins in the trunk, slurred speech, and *choreoathetosis* (uncontrolled writhing movements). Intellect is generally spared. Most children with this condition need a wheelchair for ambulation before the age of 10.

Individuals with this condition are at high risk of developing cancer, which occurs in about 38 percent of cases. The most common cancers, about 85 percent, are leukemia and lymphoma. The immune system is somewhat impaired and those affected are at risk of developing infections, especially in the lungs. They may also develop premature grey hair and endocrine abnormalities such as diabetes.

The lifespan of those with this condition has markedly improved. Most live at least into their 20s and some have survived into their 50s. The major cause of death in older individuals is lung failure.

Historical Background

The first description of the condition is an account of three siblings published in 1926 (in French) by Ladislav Syllaba, a Czech internist, and Kamil Henner, a Czech neurologist. In 1941 another case was reported in English by Denise Louis-Bar, a Belgian neurologist. For this reason, the condition is sometimes called Louis-Bar syndrome. In 1958 Elena Boder, an American physician, and Robert P. Sedgwick, an American pediatric neurologist, introduced the name *ataxia-telangiectasia*. The condition is therefore sometimes called Boder-Sedgwick syndrome as well.

Diagnosis of Condition

Ataxia-telangiectasia is suspected in children when signs of ataxia develop between the ages one and four years. It can present as a waddling gait, tilting of the head, abnormal movements of the trunk, difficulty moving eyes smoothly when following an object, and slurred speech. It is suspected more quickly when there is a family history of similar symptoms. It is further suspected when there is an elevated level of alpha-fetoprotein in the blood. It is confirmed by finding very low levels of ATM protein. When a specific mutation is known in the family or suspected in a certain ethnic group, that mutation can be tested for as well.

Genetic Cause

The gene associated with the condition is the ATM gene, which is found in the long arm of chromosome 11. It codes for the protein kinase ATM. This enzyme is important in the regulation of the response to breaks in double stranded DNA. It is for this reason that people with this condition are at higher risk for cancer, because cells in which DNA is not repaired may become cancerous. Individuals with this condition are particularly sensitive to radiation, which can break down DNA, since they lack the ability to repair these breaks. This is an important consideration in their treatment, because radiation needs to be limited.

A particular mutation is associated with those of North African Jewish descent. This mutation is called p.Arg35X.[1]

Heredity

The disease is inherited in an autosomal recessive fashion. In order to have the disease, a person must have a mutation on both copies of the gene. Carriers of one ATM mutation do not have the neurological condition but are at a fourfold risk of developing cancer, in particular breast cancer. Carrier frequency of the p.ArgX mutation in those of Moroccan and Tunisian Jewish descent is 1:80.

Living with the Condition

Physical therapy is an important component of care. The goal of the physical therapy is to minimize contractures (tightening of muscles) and scoliosis (curvature of the spine) as well as assist in appropriate adaptive equipment when needed. Speech therapy can help manage drooling, slurred speech, and feeding difficulties. Medications to control the symptoms may be of assistance in some cases.

Individuals with this condition need to be carefully monitored for early signs of cancer such as weight loss, localized pain, or bruising. If they develop cancer, it is important that they be treated in centers familiar with the management of patients with this condition, since they need to have minimal exposure to radiation and normal doses of chemotherapy can be fatal.

Individuals with this condition are at higher risk of infection, especially of the lungs and sinuses with pneumococcus. Parents should be trained in proper lung hygiene (similar to parents of children with cystic fibrosis). Affected individuals should be under the ongoing care of a pulmonologist. Giving infusions of immunoglobulins may be helpful in some cases.

Sources
R. Gatti Ataxia-Telangiectasia, GeneReviews.
http://www.ncbi.nlm.nih.gov/books/NBK26468.
S. Jozwiak, C. K. Janniger, T. Kmiec, and E. Bernatowska, eMedicine.
http://emedicine.medscape.com/article/1113394-overview.

Further Reading
Ataxia Telangiectasia. Genetics Home Reference.
http://ghr.nlm.nih.gov/condition/ataxia-telangiectasia
Ataxia-Telangiectasia. National Ataxia Foundation. www.ataxia.org/pdf/
Ataxia%20Telangiectasia.pdf

Support Organizations
AT Children's Project
5300 W. Hillsboro Blvd., #105
Coconut Creek, FL 33073
Phone: (800) 5-HELP-A-T (800.543.5728)
Fax: (954) 725-1153
Email: info@atcp.org
Internet: www.communityatcp.org
(This website includes a handbook for families.)
The National Ataxia Foundation
2600 Fernbrook Lane North, Suite 119
Minneapolis, MN 55447-4752
Phone: (763) 553-0020
Fax: (763) 553-0167
Email: naf@ataxia.org
Internet: www.ataxia.org

---

1. In codon 103 there is a point mutation, a substitution of cytosine by thiamine. This means that instead of the mRNA code reading CGA, which means arginine, it reads UGA, which means stop. The resulting protein is too short and thus less functional.

Bloom Syndrome

Summary

Children with Bloom syndrome are born very small and remain that way throughout life. They often have a red splotchy rash in sun-exposed areas, such as over the nose and cheeks (butterfly rash) and the back of the hands and forearms. They are sensitive to repeated infections, particularly of the ears and lungs. Repeated bouts of pneumonia can lead to chronic lung disease. People affected with Bloom syndrome are also likely to develop diabetes and cancer. Cancer can be of many different organs, and at more than one primary site. Cancer tends to occur at a much younger age in those affected by Bloom syndrome than in the general population and is generally the cause of death.

Historical Background

The condition was first described by Dr. David Bloom, a dermatologist, in 1954.[1] It is also sometimes called *congenital telangiectatic erythema*. Most of what is known about the syndrome comes from the Bloom Syndrome Registry, which has been maintained since 1954. As of 2004, the latest year posted on the Internet, there were 238 patients entered in the registry.

Diagnosis of Condition

Bloom syndrome is diagnosed through clinical features. Patients are born small and remain small. They tend to have a long narrow face and prominent nose. The lower jaw tends to be small, and ears tend to be large. The chromosomes themselves tend to look abnormal, with an increased number of gaps, breaks, and chromosomal rearrangements.

The syndrome is confirmed by a test in which exposure of chromosomes to bromodeoxyuridine leads to increased recombination of the chromosomes (increased exchanges between sister chromosomes). It can be further confirmed by searching for a specific genetic mutation.

Genetic Cause

The gene associated with this condition is called BLM. It is found on the long arm of chromosome 15. This gene is involved in the production of *helicases*, enzymes whose purpose is to allow the DNA to uncoil to allow proper copying. Those with a mutant BLM gene are missing this enzyme and thus repair of the DNA is inhibited and more errors can creep in during copying. This difficulty in repair is probably part of the reason for the increased susceptibility to cancer. The same phenotype is produced regardless of the mutation or combination of mutations that are found in the genotype of an affected person.

The mutation that occurs in those of Ashkenazi Jewish descent is known as BLM^{ash} (ASH is for Ashkenazi).[2]

Heredity

Bloom syndrome is inherited in an autosomal recessive manner, which means that the illness occurs only when both parents are carriers. Carrier testing is available for at-risk family members of individuals with the BLM^{ash} mutation.

Carrier frequency among Ashkenazi Jews is estimated at 1:200. Among Ashkenazi Jews of Polish descent it may be as frequent as 1:37. On the other hand, it is a very rare condition. The fact that there should be many more cases of this condition based on carrier frequency suggests that there may be incomplete penetrance—in other words, not all those who have the defective gene will develop the condition.[3]

Unaffected carriers are of normal size. There is no reason to test siblings without any signs of the syndrome. Siblings who are born small, however, should be tested.

Living with the Condition

Children with this condition require careful monitoring of caloric intake and nutritional status to help them reach their maximum growth potential. Many babies with Bloom syndrome have little interest in eating, which can also contribute to their failure to gain weight. Regurgitation and vomiting are also characteristic of this condition. If those affected have gastrointestinal reflux, it needs to be treated vigorously to prevent further weight loss.

Those with the condition, especially children, should avoid sun exposure, especially of facial skin, to prevent the red splotches that can lead to scarring. Sunlight is also a form of radiation that can increase the chances of cancer, and it should be avoided as well. Photosensitive rashes tend to improve with age.

People with this condition have lower than normal levels of immunoglobulins and tend to get more infections than normal. This situation usually improves with age, however.

Cancer is 300 times more likely to occur in patients with Bloom syndrome than in the general population, and it tends to occur at young ages. The mean age of developing leukemia is 22 years. Those who survive past this age develop solid tumors at an average age of 35 years. Therefore, care should also be taken in the use of cancer-provoking interventions such as X-rays. People with this condition also need to be monitored for development of cancer. Regular check-up and screening can help ensure that if cancer does develop it is discovered at a more treatable stage. Thus, for example, affected people should be screened for colon cancer at a much younger age than the general population. If treatment of cancer is required, different treatment regimens may need to be used.

Most reported people with Bloom syndrome are of normal intelligence. An important consideration in raising children with this syndrome is to treat them according to their chronological age, not their size.

The men who have been examined have been lacking sperm and thus appear to be infertile. No children have been born to affected men. Women with the condition may develop premature menopause. A number of such women have given birth to healthy infants, although some have delivered prematurely.

Sources
M. M. Sanz and J. German, Bloom's syndrome. GeneReviews.
http://www.ncbi.nlm.nih.gov/books/NBK1398.
A. A. Bajoghli, Bloom Syndrome, eMedicine.
http://emedicine.medscape.com/article/1110271-overview.

Further Reading
Bloom Syndrome. Genetics Home Reference.
http://ghr.nlm.nih.gov/condition/bloom-syndrome

Support Organizations
Bloom's Syndrome Foundation
7095 Hollywood Blvd, #583
Los Angeles, CA 90028
Email: info@bloomssyndrome.org
Internet: www.bloomssyndrome.org
Bloom's Connect
Email: info@bloomsconnect.org
Internet: www.bloomsconnect.org

1. D. Bloom, Congenital telangiectatic erythema resembling lupus erythematosus in dwarfs; probably a syndrome entity. AJDC 1954; 88:754–58.
2. In position 2281 of BLM cDNA, 6 base pairs are omitted, replaced by 7 base pairs. The resulting garbled message leads to a less functional protein.
3. L. E. Abel. *Jewish Genetic Disorders: A Layman's Guide.* Jefferson, NC: McFarland and Company, 2001.

Canavan Disease

Summary

Canavan disease is a degenerative neurological disease that results from the build-up of N-acetyl aspartic acid (NAA) due to the lack of the enzyme *aspartoacylase*. The lack of this enzyme leads to destruction of the white matter of the brain, making it look spongy on pathological examination. Another name of the disease is "spongy degeneration of the brain." White matter of the brain is largely made up of myelin, a fatty covering of the nerve sheaths. Therefore, Canavan disease is considered one of the leukodystrophies, diseases of the myelin.

Infants with this condition are normal at birth but by three to five months have developed large heads and very low muscle tone. They fail to reach motor developmental milestones such as sitting, standing, and speech. However, they do show reactions to their surroundings, such as smiling and laughing. Vision is generally present at first and may later be lost. Hearing is generally intact. Over time they become very spastic, or stiff, and may develop seizures. Feeding becomes more difficult. While there are descriptions of a number of forms of the disease (neonatal, infantile, and late onset), it is most likely that there is only one disease and that it has variable progression. Length of survival depends on the severity of the condition and on medical care received. However, those with this condition rarely live beyond the teenage years.

Historical Background

In 1931 Dr. Myrtelle May Moore Canavan published a paper describing the autopsy of a child who had died at 16 months and whose brain had a spongy white section. This was the first description of this degenerative disorder of the central nervous system, and the condition came to bear her name.

Diagnosis of Condition

The condition is suspected in infants who have large heads and are hypotonic. Around the age of three to five months, when they are lifted by their hands, their heads will lean backward, a finding known as "head lag." In normal development, head lag is expected to disappear by three months.

The disease is diagnosed by measurement of the concentration of NAA in the urine, where it is found to be much higher than that of normal controls. The lack of activity of aspartoacylase (the enzyme that breaks down NAA) can be shown in cultures of skin cells (fibroblasts) as well.

Genetic Cause

The gene associated with Canavan disease is known as ASPA. This gene, located on chromosome 17, codes for the enzyme aspartoacylase. Lack of this enzyme causes build-up of NAA and loss of the myelin sheath that enables nerve conduction, and leads to the sponginess described above.

In persons of Ashkenazi Jewish descent, the disease is usually (98 percent of the time) caused by one of two mutations.[1]

Heredity

Canavan disease is an autosomal disease; to be affected, a child must inherit a defective copy of the gene from both parents. Carriers of the disease are not at risk of getting the disorder.

The frequency of carrying any mutation of the ASPA gene in those of Ashkenazi Jewish descent is estimated at between one in 40 and one in 60.

Living with the Condition

Physical and intellectual decline continues throughout the lifespan. Independent sitting, walking, and speech are generally not achieved. However, steps can be taken to improve the ease of care. For example, physical therapy can help minimize contractures (tightening of muscles) and improve tone and positioning. Speech therapy can help provide alternate methods of communication and help assess feeding ability. As feeding becomes more difficult, placement of a gastrostomy tube (feeding tube) can help maintain adequate nutrition and minimize chances of aspiration.

Sources

R. Matalon and G. Bhatia, Canavan Disease. GeneReviews. http://www.ncbi.nlm.nih.gov/books/NBK1234/

Further Reading

Canavan Disease Information Page. www.ninds.nih.gov/disorders/canavan/canavan.htm
Canavan Disease. Genetics Home Reference. http://ghr.nlm.nih.gov/condition/canavan-disease

Support Organizations
Canavan Foundation
450 West End Avenue, #6A
New York, NY 10024
Phone: (877) 4-CANAVAN
Fax: (212) 873-7892
Email: info@canavanfoundation.org
Internet: www.canavanfoundation.org

This organization has a rabbinic advisory committee.
Canavan Research Foundation
88 Route 37
New Fairfield, CT 06812
Phone: (203) 746-2436
Fax: (203) 746-3205
Email: info@canavan.org
Internet: http://www.canavan.org
Canavan Disease Research
PO Box 8194
Rolling Meadows, IL 60008-8194
Phone: (800) 833-2194
Email: info@canavanresearch.org
Internet: www.canavanresearch.org
United Leukodystrophy Foundation
2304 Highland Drive
Sycamore, IL 60178
Phone: (815) 895-3211; (800) 728-5483
Fax: (815) 895-2432
Email: office@ulf.org
Internet: www.ulf.org
National Tay-Sachs and Allied Diseases Association
2001 Beacon Street
Suite 204
Boston, MA 02135
Phone: (800) 90NTSAD (906-8723)
Fax: (617) 277-1034
Email: info@ntsad.org
Internet: www.ntsad.org

1. One of these is p.Glu285Ala. In this mutation, glutamine at position 285 is replaced by alanine. The other is pTyr231X, where a stop codon occurs instead of the code for tyrosine. These mutations occur in 3 percent of cases in the non-Jewish population. An additional 1 percent of Jewish cases are caused by the mutation that causes 40–60 percent of non-Jewish cases, a mutation known as pAla305Glu. In that mutation, glutamine replaces alanine at position 305.

Congenital Adrenal Hyperplasia

Introduction

Congenital Adrenal Hyperplasia (CAH) is a condition in which a lack of enzymes in the adrenal glands leads to the inability to make an important steroid called *cortisol*. There are a number of types of CAH, two of which are associated with Jewish ancestry. In the more common condition, **CAH I**, the enzyme 21 hydroxylase is not produced. In another version, **CAH IV**, the missing enzyme is 11-β hydroxylase. In both conditions, the pituitary gland responds to the lack of cortisol by stimulating the adrenals to keep trying to produce it. This leads to build-up of other steroids[1] along the pathway. Symptoms include varying degrees of virilization (the accruement of male sexual characteristics) in girls, and potentially life-threatening loss of salts (such as sodium) in both sexes.

Congenital Adrenal Hyperplasia I – 21 Hydroxylase Deficiency, Late Onset

Summary

Congenital adrenal hyperplasia I (CAH I) can be either classic or nonclassic. The classic form is very similar to CAH IV (see below). Symptoms include loss of salts, girls being born with ambiguous genitalia, and early growth. These are discussed in detail in the section on CAH IV. In the nonclassic form of CAH I, which is more common in those of Ashkenazi Jewish descent, there is only a moderate enzyme deficiency. These individuals are not born with ambiguous genitalia, but girls later in life can present with signs of virilization (the effects of male hormones). Other effects include acne and hairiness. Women with this condition tend to have irregular periods, which are sometimes the only sign of the condition.

Historical Background

The high frequency of nonclassic CAH I in the Jewish population has been noted since 1985.[2]

Diagnosis of Condition

The condition is suspected in girls with heavy body hair or irregular menses. These symptoms are similar to polycystic ovary syndrome (PCOS).[3] Due to the high frequency of the mutation for CAH in the Ashkenazi Jewish community, testing for CAH should be considered in women with presumed PCOS. CAH is also suspected in cases of infertility. In boys, it may be suspected if hairiness develops at a younger than expected age. Mild cases are most likely to be undetected in boys. CAH I is confirmed by the presence of elevated levels of 17 hydroxyprogesterone, the substance in the cortisol pathway on which the defective enzyme is meant to work. Targeted genetic mutation analysis can then be performed.

Genetic Cause

21 hydroxylase deficiency CAH is caused by mutations in the CYP21A2 (also known as CYP21B) gene located on the short arm of chromosome 6. This mutation leads to a defective 21 hydroxylase enzyme.

The mutation most common among those of Ashkenazi Jewish descent is V281L.[4] Affected persons either are generally homozygous for this mutation or have this mutation in combination with another mutation (compound heterozygous). Those with the V281L mutation almost always have the nonclassic form of the condition.[5]

Heredity

CAH I is inherited in an autosomal recessive fashion. Therefore, a defective gene must be inherited from both parents in order for a child to have the condition.

The carrier frequency in the Ashkenazi Jewish population is approximately 1:5.

Living with the Condition

Many people with nonclassic CAH I are asymptomatic. Women with symptoms of excess hair, irregular menses, and/or infertility can be treated with oral steroids.

The symptoms of and treatment for classic CAH are similar to those of CAH IV, which are discussed below.

Congenital Adrenal Hyperplasia IV – 11β Hydroxylase Deficiency
Summary

In CAH IV, and also in the classic form of CAH I, the excess steroids that build up cause virilization—the accruement of male sexual characteristics. Affected girls are born with ambiguous genitalia—external organs that resemble those of boys although they have functional female internal organs (ovaries and uterus). Boys affected by this condition begin to show signs of puberty starting at a very young age (such as 2–4 years). Children with this condition will also grow fast and be tall for their age. However, especially if the condition is untreated, the growth plates in the bones will fuse earlier and their final adult height will be shorter than expected.

In some cases (known as "saltwasters"), the lack of the enzymes can also lead to lack of steroids that are needed for the control of salt balance. This lack of control, in severe cases, can be life-threatening. Patients with CAH IV also have a high incidence of high blood pressure.

Historical Background

Congenital adrenal hyperplasia has probably existed since antiquity. The Talmud contains many discussions about the "androgynos"—someone who has both male and female external genitalia. It is likely that at least some of these people had congenital adrenal hyperplasia.

Diagnosis of Condition

The condition is suspected in female infants born with ambiguous genitalia or in boys who develop body hair at a very early age. Confirmation in both genders is done through checking levels of steroids in the blood. In CAH IV the levels of 11 deoxycortisol will be markedly elevated. In communities where a particular mutation is common, or in families with a known genetic mutation, the mutation can be tested for directly.

Genetic Cause

The condition is caused by mutations in the CYP11B1 gene found on the long arm of chromosome 8. The mutation that is common in those of Moroccan Jewish descent is called R448H.[6]

Heredity

This condition is inherited in an autosomal recessive fashion. In order to have the condition, a mutation has to be inherited from both parents.

The carrier rate of the R448H mutation in the overall Moroccan Jewish community appears to be 1:188. In earlier studies of families who lived in the Atlas Mountains, the carrier frequency was between 1:35 and 1:42.

Living with the Condition[7]

Once the diagnosis is made, the symptoms of salt-wasting can be kept under control with use of medicinal steroids, which give the pituitary the feedback it needs to stop overstimulating the adrenal glands. These medications are generally given twice daily by mouth. External steroids, however, have a number of side effects (including build-up of fat in particular parts of the body and puffy cheeks, an appearance that is known as *Cushingoid*). The external steroids can also suppress the adrenals so they cannot respond in a normal fashion at times of stress (e.g., infections, surgery, trauma). Therefore, consultation with an endocrinologist is important to find the appropriate balance of medication. Families also need to be educated regarding situations (e.g., illness, surgery) where the dose needs to be adjusted.

It is more difficult to deal with virilization that has already happened, especially in genetic females. Surgery can correct the external ambiguous genitalia to resemble more normal female anatomy. However, the vaginal opening that is created will not always have the expandability of a natural vagina, leading to less pleasant marital relations. At times the surgery impairs the capacity for sensation in the genital area, which also affects enjoyment of marital relations. There has been much debate about this surgery. On the one hand, if it is performed in infancy, the child can be brought up with a clear gender. On the other hand, it prevents the child from having a say in this decision, which will affect her for life. Since the gender that a child is raised has halachic considerations (see chapter on ambiguous genitalia), rabbinic advice should be sought as part of the decision making process.

Giving steroids to the mother during pregnancy has been shown to reduce the virilization of the female fetus. In order to be effective, it needs to be started at 4–5 weeks of pregnancy, before the mother knows if she is carrying a boy or a girl or whether the fetus has inherited the genetic mutation. The treatment is stopped if chorionic villi sampling or amniocentesis shows that the fetus is a boy, or a girl who does not have the genetic mutation. This treatment will not prevent other symptoms of the condition, only the ambiguous genitalia. Boys with the condition will start steroids at a later age. Prenatal treatment is still subject to controversy, because its long-term consequences are not yet known.

Sources
Congenital Adrenal Hyperplasia – 21 Hydroxylase Deficiency, Late Onset
S. Nimkarn, M.I. New, 21-Hydroxylase-Deficient Congenital Adrenal Hyperplasia. GeneReviews.
http://www.ncbi.nlm.nih.gov/books/NBK1171/
R. C. Wilson, S. Nimkarn, M. Dumic, et al., Ethnic Specific Distribution

of Mutations in 716 Patients with Congenital Adrenal Hyperplasia Owing to 21-Hydroxylase Deficiency. *Mol Genet Metab.* 2007 April: 90(4): 414–21.

Congenital Adrenal Hyperplasia IV – 11β Hydroxylase Deficiency
Uwaifo GI. C-11 Hydroxylase Deficiency. eMedicine.
http://emedicine.medscape.com/article/117012-overview
T. Paperna, R. Gershoni-Baruch, K. Badarneh, L. Kasinetz and Z. Hochberg, Mutations in CYP11B1 and Congenital Adrenal Hyperplasia in Moroccan Jews. *J. Clin. Endocrinol. Metab.* 2005, 90:5463–65.

Further Reading
NIH Fact Sheet, Congenital Adrenal Hyperplasia. http://www.cc.nih.gov/ccc/patient_education/pepubs/cah.pdf

A full book on CAH for parents has been published as well:
C. Y. Hsu, S. A. Rivkees. *Congenital Adrenal Hyperplasia: A Parents' Guide.* CHSR Enterprises, LLC, 2005.

Support Organizations
CARES Foundation
2414 Morris Aveue, Suite 110
Union, NJ 07083
Phone: (866) 227-3737
Email: contact@caresfoundation.org
Internet: www.caresfoundation.org
CAH Support Group
2 Windrush Close
Flitwick, Bedfordshire MK45 1PX
Support Helpline: 015257 717536
Internet: www.livingwithcah.com

---

1. In CAH I, these include 17 hydroxyprogesterone, delta 4 androstenedione, and progesterone. In CAH IV, 11 deoxycortisol is one of the steroids that builds up.
2. W. P. Speiser, B. Dupont, P. Rubinstein, A. Piazza, A. Kastelan, and M. I. New. High frequency of non-classical steroid 21 hydroxylase deficiency. *An J Hum Genet.* 1985; 37:650–67.

3. An endocrine disorder that is one of the most common causes of infertility. The classic symptoms include obesity, irregular menses due to lack of ovulation, and signs of male hormones such as extra facial hair and acne. Typical findings of cysts on ultrasound of the ovaries is what gives the syndrome its name. It is possible to have the condition without exhibiting all of the symptoms.

4. In codon 844, guanine is replaced by thiamine. As a result, the DNA codes for leucine instead of valine at the 281 (or 282) position. At times this mutation is known as V282L as the numbering nomenclature has changed over time.

5. Less than 3 percent with a genotype assumed to lead to the nonclassic form will in fact have the classic phenotype.

6. In codon 448 of the DNA, guanine is replaced by adenine. In the resulting protein, arginine is replaced by histidine. This protein is the enzyme 11-β hydroxylase, the enzyme that breaks down deoxycorticosterone to corticosterone.

7. The information in this section applies to both CAH IV and to the classic form of CAH I.

Costeff Syndrome

Summary

Costeff syndrome is a condition in which there is lack of development of the optic nerve in both eyes, associated with a disorder of uncontrolled movements known as *chorea*. It starts before age 10 and progresses slowly, generally stabilizing in the second decade of life. Some people with the condition develop progressive paralysis or spasticity (tight muscles). Some develop mild intellectual impairment in the teenage years, although they are generally able to complete school despite the difficulties. Speech difficulties such as a nasal voice are common; swallowing difficulties are rare. The degree to which individuals who have the mutation causing this disease are affected is varied, even in the same family.

The disease is a form of 3 methylglutaconic aciduria (3MGA), known as 3MGA Type III. Persons with the defect have an impairment of the body's ability to make energy in mitochondria, the energy-producing subunits of the cell. This leads to the neurological symptoms. In addition, as a result of this deficiency, large amounts of 3 methylglutaconic acid, a breakdown product of the amino acid leucine, build up and are excreted in the urine; this is tested for in the diagnosis of the condition.

Historical Background

This condition was described in 1989 by Dr. Hanan Costeff, an Israeli neurologist. The association with a defect in the OPA3 gene was reported in 2001.

Diagnosis of Condition

The disease is suspected in those with visual difficulty and movement disorders. Elevated levels of 3 methylglutaconic acid and 3 methylglutaric acid in the urine make the diagnosis likely. Finding a deficit in the gene OPA3 confirms the diagnosis. In the Iraqi Jewish population, this can be done by targeted mutation analysis for the mutation unique to this population.

Genetic Cause

The mutation is in the OPA3 gene, which is found on chromosome 19. This gene provides instructions for making a protein that is found in mitochondria but whose exact function is not yet known.

Heredity

The disease is inherited in an autosomal recessive fashion. To be affected, a person needs to inherit the defective OPA3 gene from both parents.

This condition occurs in Jews of Iraqi origin. The mutation in this population is called c143-1G>C.[1] In a group that originated from Baghdad, the carrier frequency of this mutation was 1:10.

Living with the Condition

Proper educational assistance with needed modifications for the visual difficulty is important. The degree to which a person is affected is variable. Many may become legally blind. Getting training for reduced vision while one can still see is helpful in learning how to adapt. Ongoing monitoring by an ophthalmologist can help prevent further vision loss from any other reversible causes.

The difficulties in vocalization can be helped by a speech therapist. Occupational and physical therapists can help deal with the difficulties presented by the lack of balance and paralysis that may set in. The degree of help that will be needed will depend on the degree to which a person is affected by the condition, since the amount of deterioration can vary from needing minimal assistance to requiring a wheelchair.

Sources

M. Gunay-Aygun, W. A. Gahl, and Y. Anikster, 3 Methylglutaconic Aciduria Type 3. GeneReviews.
http://www.ncbi.nlm.nih.gov/books/NBK1473

Y. Anikster, R. Kleta, A. Shaag, W. A. Gah, and O. Elpeleg. Type III 3 Methylglutaconic Aciduria (Optic Atrophy Plus Syndrome, or Costeff Optic Atrophy Syndrome): Identification of the OPA3 Gene and its Founder Mutation in Iraqi Jews. *Am. J. Hum. Genet.* 69:1218–24, 2001.

Costeff Syndrome (3 methylglutaconic acid) [Hebrew]. *Israeli Journal of Neurology.*
Available online at www.medicalmedia.co.il/publications/ArticleDetails. aspx?artid=2259&sheetid=161

Suggested Reading

3 Methylglutaconic aciduria type III. Genetics Home Reference.
http://ghr.nlm.nih.gov/condition/3-methylglutaconic-aciduria

Support Organizations
Organic Acidemia Association
Carol Barton, Executive Director
PO. Box 1008
Pinole, CA 94564
Phone: (510) 672-2476
Fax (toll free): (866) 539-4060
Email: carolbarton@oaanews.org
Internet: www.oaanews.org
CLIMB — Children Living with Inherited Metabolic Diseases
Climb Building
176 Nantwich Road
Crewe CW2 6BG
Phone: 0800 652 3181
Fax: 0845 241 2174
Email: fam.svcs@climb.org.uk
Internet: www.climb.org.uk

---

1. The type of mutation is a *splice mutation*. This means that the mutation is exactly at the point where introns (those parts of the DNA that are not expressed) are meant to be removed in the final processing of messenger RNA. With a mutation at this point, the information of the intron is left in the final protein produced, which is therefore less functional.

Cystic Fibrosis

Summary

Cystic fibrosis is a condition affecting cell membranes, in which cells expel too little chloride and absorb too much sodium and water. The lack of water outside the cells leads to the production of very thick mucus. This mucus can plug up airways of the lungs and thus lead to difficulty breathing and/or chronic inflammation and infection. The mucus can also plug the pancreas and prevent the proper digestion of foods, especially fats. The mucus can affect the sweat glands so there may be excessive salt on the skin, which may cause the skin to taste salty.

The most dangerous aspect of cystic fibrosis is generally the lung disease. Plugged airways lead to difficulty breathing, and lack of proper airway drainage increases the chances of infection. Repeated episodes of infection can damage lung tissue and lead to chronic lung disease. The most common cause of death is end-stage lung disease.

Improper digestion can lead to vitamin deficiencies and difficulty in growth. It can also interfere with the functioning of the immune system, leading to infections. Plugging of the intestines by thick secretions can lead to a form of intestinal obstruction in newborns known as *meconium ileus*.

Historical Background

Dr. Dorothy Andersen, the pathologist at New York Babies Hospital, noticed that a number of children who had cystic findings in their pancreas on autopsy had a similar clinical picture, consisting of an intestine plugged with meconium, and respiratory and gastrointestinal problems. She published her findings in 1938. She concluded that this was a genetic disease inherited in an autosomal recessive manner. A few years later, Dr. Sydney Farber described the generalized nature of the condition and coined the term *mucoviscidosis*.[1]

Diagnosis of Condition

In about 15 to 20 percent of affected infants, the disease presents as meconium ileus. Beyond the newborn stage, it is suspected when a child has repeated episodes of lung disease such as pneumonia, or has significant difficulty gaining weight (failure to thrive). Very mild cases may not be picked up until adulthood as part of a workup for male infertility. Currently, screening for cystic fibrosis is one of the routine blood tests performed on newborns in the hospital in many countries (including the U.S. and Israel). This is a screening test; if an elevated level of immunoreactive trypsinogen (IRT), an enzyme created by the pancreas, is found, the test needs to either be repeated or confirmed with additional testing. As there has been much debate about the proper method of mass diagnosis and screening for this condition, official guidelines have been published as to the proper diagnosis of cystic fibrosis.[2]

Genetic Cause
The disease is caused by one of over 1,600 possible mutations in the gene for *cystic fibrosis transmembrane conductance regular* (CFTR). This gene, found on chromosome 7, codes for a protein whose purpose is to allow the excretion of chloride from cells.

There is great variation in the degree to which people with the same genotype are affected. There is some correlation between genotype and pancreatic function phenotype. The genotypes that occur most commonly in Ashkenazi Jews are more likely to cause pancreatic dysfunction. In contrast, there has not been shown to be a correlation between type of mutation and lung disease. Environmental factors such as exposure to cigarette smoke and frequency of infections seem to play a large role in the degree of lung disease.[3]

Heredity
The disease is inherited in an autosomal recessive manner. To have the disease, a mutation has to be inherited from both parents. In some cases, the child can be affected by inheriting different mutations of the gene from each parent.

Cystic fibrosis has been reported in all ethnic groups but is most common in those of white European ancestry. One in 29 people of eastern European origin is a carrier of a CFTR mutation. Seventy percent of these will have one particular mutation known as Delta F 508.[4] The rate in Ashkenazi Jews is similar to that of non-Jews from the same areas. However, the groups tend to have different distributions of mutations. In Ashkenazi Jews, Delta F 508 accounts for 23 percent and W1282x (an otherwise rare mutation) accounts for 60 percent. An additional 4 percent of cases are caused by G542x. The remaining percentage have an assortment of other mutations.

Screening of the healthy population in Israel has shown that many non-Ashkenazi Jews are carriers as well. The prevalence of cystic fibrosis mutations was 1:19, 1:28, and 1:42 for those whose grandparents were of Sephardi (Spain, Holland, Greece, Italy, Israel), North African (Morocco, Libya, Tunisia, Egypt), and Eastern (Iran, Iraq, India, Georgia, Bulgaria) origin, respectively. This study tested for a panel of 12 mutations. A more recent study of patients with cystic fibrosis found 15 mutations that occurred in more than one patient, with variation as to the specific mutation among ethnic groups. Therefore, in cases of inter-ethnic marriage, it is important to get specific counseling for screening for this condition and not just rely on the standard Ashkenazi panel.[5]

Living with the Condition

Care of the pulmonary component of the disease generally involves a combination of treatment and prevention of pulmonary complications. This is done by helping the person move the thickened secretion with some form of chest physical therapy. This can involve manual physical therapy ("clapping"), special vibration vests, physical activity, or a combination thereof. Affected people are generally treated with bronchodilators by inhaler or nebulizer and by antibiotics.

Nutritional difficulties are generally managed with a combination of high-calorie diet and oral replacement of pancreatic enzymes. Special attention has to be taken to assure adequate supply of fat-soluble vitamins (A, D, E, K) and zinc. At times, special formulas may be needed to assure adequate nutrition. A nutritionist is usually part of the care team.

The care of children with cystic fibrosis has advanced markedly. In the past, this disease was generally fatal in childhood. Now, with careful pulmonary care and attention to proper nutrition, the mean age of survival is 37 years. Multidisciplinary care in a Cystic Fibrosis Center has been shown to increase survival. With continued advances in knowledge as to the best methods of care, life expectancy is continuing to rise. Mild cases are also possible. Therefore, if a child is diagnosed with cystic fibrosis, the mother and the apparently healthy siblings should be tested as well. Even if there are no obvious symptoms, a diagnosis of cystic fibrosis will ensure the lung and nutritional care needed to maintain good health.

A number of children have been born to mothers who have cystic fibrosis. The mother's health needs to be taken into consideration. Prognosis is good in those with mild to moderate disease. Males with cystic fibrosis are infertile 95 percent of the time due to lack of development or atrophy of the system needed for transfer of sperm. They do, however, produce sperm in the testes. Therefore, fatherhood by artificial reproductive technology is a possibility.

Sources
G. Sharma, Cystic Fibrosis. eMedicine.
http://emedicine.medscape.com/article/1001602-overview
S. M. Moskowitz, J. F. Chmiel, et al. CFTR-Related Disorders.
GeneReviews.
http://www.ncbi.nlm.nih.gov/books/NBK1250/
E. L. Abel, *Jewish Genetic Disorders*. Jefferson, NC: Macfarland and Co.,
2001.

Further Reading
Cystic Fibrosis. *MedlinePlus Encyclopedia.* http://www.nlm.nih.gov/
medlineplus/ency/article/000107.htm
Cystic Fibrosis. Genetics Home Reference.
http://ghr.nlm.nih.gov/condition/cystic-fibrosis
KidsHealth from Nemours.
http://kidshealth.org/

Support Organizations
Cystic Fibrosis Foundation
United States
Cystic Fibrosis Foundation (national headquarters)
6931 Arlington Road, 2nd Floor
Bethesda, MD 20814
Phone: (301) 951-4422, (800) FIGHT CF (344-4823)
Fax: (301) 951-6378
Email: info@cff.org
Internet: www.cff.org
Israel
Igud Cystic Fibrosis
Krinitzy 79
Ramat Gan 52423
Phone: (03) 670-2323
Fax: (03) 670-2324
Email: cd@cff.org.il
Internet: www.cff.org.il

Cystic Fibrosis Trust
11 London Road Bromley Kent BR1 1BY
Phone: 020 8464 7211
Fax: 020 8313 0472
Email: enquiries@cftrust.org.uk, for general enquiries
Email: AskTheExpert@cftrust.org.uk, for medical enquiries
Internet: www.cftrust.org.uk

---

1. For a complete review of the historical development of the diagnosis and treatment of this condition, see Littlewood, J. Looking back over 40 years and what the future holds. Available at http://www.cftrust.org.uk/aboutcf/whatiscf/cfhistory/Levy_Lecture_04_-_JL.pdf.

2. P. M. Farrell, B. J. Rosenstein, T. B. White, et al. Guidelines for Diagnosis of Cystic Fibrosis in Newborns through Older Adults: Cystic Fibrosis Foundation Consensus Report. *J Pediatr* 2008; 153:S4–S14.

3. D. Langfelder-Schwind, E. Kloza, E. Sugarman, et al. Cystic fibrosis prenatal screening in genetic counseling practice: recommendations of the National Society of Genetic Counselors. *Journal Genetic Counseling* 2005; 14:1–15.

4. A deletion of phenylalanine at positive 508.

5. A. Quint, I. Lerer, M. Sagi, and D. Abeliovich. Mutation Spectrum in Jewish Cystic Fibrosis Patients in Israel: Implication to Carrier Screening. *Am J Med Gen* 2005; 136A: 246–248.

Dubin-Johnson Syndrome

Summary
Dubin Johnson syndrome is a condition in which there are elevated levels of bilirubin. This can appear as jaundice, in which the skin and the whites of the eyes look yellow. The type of bilirubin that is elevated is known as direct, or conjugated, bilirubin. Other than the jaundice, the clinical course of the condition is relatively mild. It is important to recognize, however, in order to prevent multiple tests looking for other causes of the symptom.

Historical Background
The condition was first described in 1954 by Drs. I. N. Dubin and F. B. Johnson.

Diagnosis of Condition
The condition is suspected when there is elevated direct bilirubin combined with otherwise normal liver tests. It is confirmed by finding a unique pattern of breakdown products of red blood cells in the urine. In certain ethnic groups, particular mutations can be tested for.

Genetic Cause
The gene associated with the condition is the MRP2 (or ABCC2) gene found on the long arm of chromosome 10. This gene codes for the multidrug resistance protein 2 (MRP2), which helps transport certain chemicals across the liver cell membrane. The impaired transport appears to be related to the accumulation of elevated levels of bilirubin and black pigment in the liver cells.

The mutation that is common in those of Iranian Jewish descent is I1173F.[1] Those of Moroccan Jewish descent have a different mutation, known as R1150H.[2]

Heredity
Dubin Johnson syndrome is inherited in an autosomal recessive manner. Thus, in order to have the condition one has to inherit a mutation from both parents. The carrier rate of the I117F mutation in the Iranian Jewish community is 1:20 and the carrier rate of the R1150H mutation in the Moroccan Jewish community is 1:100.

Living with the Condition
Most patients are asymptomatic other than jaundice. The jaundice is generally not itchy and does not need treatment. Jaundice can be more prominent during pregnancy and if taking hormonal contraception.

Sources
S. L. Habashi, L. R. Lambiase, M. K. Anand, K. J. Mishar, and C. Nguyen. Dubin Johnson Syndrome. eMedicine Gastroenterology. http://emedicine.medscape.com/article/173517-overview
S. S. Rabinowitz, H. Elkhidi, M. S. Carter, and S. Gross. Dubin Johnson Syndrome. eMedicine Pediatrics. http://emedicine/medscape/com/article/928711-overview

Suggested Reading
Dubin Johnson Syndrome. Genetics Home Reference. http://ghr.nlm.nih.gov/condition/dubin-johnson-syndrome

Support Organizations
American Liver Foundation
75 Maiden Lane, Suite 603
New York, NY 10038
Phone: (212) 668-1000
Phone: (800) 465-4837
Fax: (212) 483-8179
Email: info@liverfoundation.org
Internet: http://www.liverfoundation.org
NIH/National Digestive Diseases Information Clearinghouse
2 Information Way
Bethesda, MD 20892-3570
Phone: (800) 891-5389
Fax: (301) 907-8906
Email: nddic@info.niddk.nih.gov
Internet: www2.niddk.nih.gov

---

1. Because of a switch in the genetic code of thymine instead of adenine, isoleucine is replaced by phenylalanine at position 1173.
2. Because of a switch in the DNA code of cysteine instead of alanine, the amino acid arginine is replaced by histidine.

Factor Deficiencies

Blood contains a number of components that cooperate to cause clotting when it is necessary to stop bleeding. One component is the platelets, a type of blood cell.[1] The other components are a series of molecules that work together and are known individually as *factors*. Defects in certain factors have been associated with certain Jewish ancestries. Bleeding disorders have been recognized from antiquity and are hinted at in the Talmud.

Factor VII Deficiency
Summary

Factor VII is a protein that is needed for proper blood clotting. A reduced level of this factor in the blood can lead to spontaneous bleeding, particularly into the joints, muscles, brain, or spinal cord. In women, it can also lead to excessive bleeding during menses. People with this condition are likely to have many nosebleeds, bleeding from gums, blood in stool or vomit, and easy bruising. They may bleed longer than normal during surgery or after injury. The severity of bleeding is variable, even within families, and does not necessarily correlate with the level of Factor VII in the blood.

Historical Background

The existence of Factor VII and its role in the clotting mechanism was discovered in 1951. The molecular basis for the deficiency in Moroccan and Iranian Jews was reported in 1996.

Diagnosis of Condition

The condition is suspected when there are bleeding episodes in the first few months of life, often prolonged bleeding after a circumcision. It is also suspected when there are abnormal results on tests for clotting, which are sometimes done before surgery.[2] It can be confirmed by measurement of levels of Factor VII. In those with a known family mutation or from certain ethnic groups, it can be further confirmed by genetic mutation analysis.

Genetic Cause

Factor VII deficiency is caused by mutations in the F7 gene found on the long arm of chromosome 13. The mutations lead to low levels of Factor VII, whose role is to combine with tissue factor to begin the sequence that leads to proper blood clotting. A specific mutation, Ala244Val,[3] is found in Jewish patients with this condition from Morocco and Iran.

Heredity

The condition is inherited in an autosomal recessive manner. To have the condition, one needs to inherit a mutation from both parents. The carrier rate of the Ala244Val mutation in those from Morocco is 1:42 and in those from Iran is 1:40.

Factor XI Deficiency
Summary

Factor XI is a protein that is needed for proper blood clotting. A reduced level of this factor in the blood can lead to excessive bleeding, particularly after surgery or significant injury. In women, it can also lead to excessive bleeding during menses. The disease that results from deficiency of this factor is also called PTA (for Plasma Thromboplastin Antecedent) deficiency, Rosenthal syndrome, or hemophilia C.

The amount of bleeding among those with reduced Factor XI is variable. Even within the same family, some patients will be affected more severely than others. People with activity levels less than 15 percent of normally functioning Factor XI are likely to have mild to moderate bleeding—usually after some trigger such as circumcision, tooth extraction, menses, or surgery. They rarely bleed spontaneously into joints or soft tissues in the manner seen in hemophilia A or B. People with activity levels of 15–70 percent normally functioning Factor XI will tend to bleed excessively only after serious injury or surgery.

Historical Background

This bleeding disorder was first described in 1953 when Dr. R. Rosenthal and others described prolonged bleeding in two sisters after dental surgery.[4]

Diagnosis of Condition

The condition is suspected in cases of prolonged bleeding such as may occur after circumcision or a surgical procedure. A clotting disorder may be suspected after routine preoperative screening, with further evaluation leading to the diagnosis. Because carriage of a mutation in this gene is rather frequent, and because even those who carry only one abnormal gene can at times be affected by surgery, there are those who recommend that all Ashkenazi Jews be tested for blood clotting ability prior to elective surgery.[5] However, this is not standard practice at present and thus each individual should discuss this matter with his or her physician. Those who are known to have the mutation should certainly notify their physicians so that potential bleeding difficulties can be properly prepared for. Those with a known family history of this condition should probably be tested, since it can impact on their own health care.

Genetic Cause

Factor XI Deficiency is generally caused by one of a number of mutations in a gene on the long arm of chromosome 4. Two particular mutations, known as Type II[6] and Type III,[7] are common among those of Jewish descent. Most commonly, defects in this gene result in reduced levels of Factor XI. Occasionally the amount produced is normal but the protein does not function normally.

Heredity

Very low levels are seen primarily in those who inherit a mutation from each parent. Thus this disease is generally defined as an autosomal recessive disease. However, heterozygotes, those who inherit only one abnormal copy of the gene, can have levels in the range of 50–70 percent and show clinical symptoms after surgery. The carrier frequency is estimated to be between 1:10 and 1:20 in the Ashkenazi Jewish population.

While this condition is most common in those of Ashkenazi Jewish descent, the Type II mutation has also been found with similar frequency among Jews of Iraqi descent. Since this population is believed to have lived in Iraq since the Babylonian Exile in about 586 BCE. (Babylon is located in present-day Iraq), it is probable that the mutation already existed in Jews at that time. The mutation that occurs only in Ashkenazi Jews is likely to have developed later, after the migration of Jews to Western countries.[8] [9]

Living with the Condition

Factor VII Deficiency is the more severe condition. Individuals with the condition need to minimize injury to those areas likely to bleed. Contact sports should be avoided. Sports that put strain on the knees should be minimized as well. Keeping fit, however, is important, because strong muscles lessen the frequency of bleeding into joints. Swimming is often the best sport. Those with the condition and their families need to be aware of the symptoms of potentially life-threatening bleeding into locations such as the head, neck area, and spine, and should seek immediate medical care if necessary.

Bleeding from a factor deficiency can generally be brought under control with a number of different treatments. These treatments are considered for procedures where bleeding is expected, such as *brit milah*, childbirth, or surgery. Consultation with a hematologist before such procedures is recommended.

Factor VII Deficiency

Bleeding into muscles and joints can generally be handled at home with rest, elevation of the limb, compression of the bleeding area, and application of ice. In the case of more severe bleeds, or before surgery, Factor VII has to be replaced. Blood products that contain Factor VII can be used in an emergency. Factor VII that is produced in the laboratory (recombinant Factor VII) is available and minimizes the risk of blood-borne diseases. For some bleeding situations, other, non-blood product medications known as *anti-fibrinolytics* can be used. These medications help hold a clot in place once it has formed by preventing its breakdown.

Factor XI Deficiency

Donated Factor XI can be used when needed to prevent bleeding as outlined below. This factor can be found in the liquid component of blood, known as the plasma. In the Unites States, the donated factor is given via a form of plasma known as *fresh frozen plasma*. In some other countries such as the United Kingdom, a product that concentrates the Factor XI is available. Because these are blood products, they carry the risk of transmitted viral infections such as hepatitis C and thus are used only when truly needed to stop or prevent bleeding. For some bleeding situations, other, anti-fibrinolytics can be used (see previous paragraph). For dental extractions, a product known as *fibrin glue* (developed in Israel) can also be of help.

Sources
Factor VII
H. Hartung, Factor VII deficiency. eMedicine Pediatrics.
http://emedicine.medscape.com/article/960592-overview

J. Ramanarayanan, G. S. Krishnan, and F. J. Hernandez-Ilizaliturri, Factor VII. eMedicine Hematology.
http://emedicine.medscape.com/article/209585-overview
M. Giansily-Blaizot, Inherited factor VII deficiency. Orphanet Encyclopedia. www.orpha.net/data/patho/GB/uk-factorVII.pdf
H. Tamary, Y. Fromovich, L. Shalmon, et al., Ala244Val is a common, probably ancient mutation causing factor VII deficiency in Moroccan and Iranian Jews. *Thromb Haemost.* 1996; 76:283–91.

Factor XI
J. E. Siegal, Factor XI deficiency. eMedicine.
http://emedicine.medscape.com/article/209984-overview
F XI Deficiency Mutation Database
www.factorxi.org
R. Asakai, D. W. Chung, E. S. Davie, and U. Seligsohn, Factor XI deficiency in Ashkenazi Jews in Israel. *N Eng J Med* 1991; 325:153–58.

Further Reading
National Hemophilia Organization, www.hemophilia.org/NHFWeb/
MainPgs/MainNHF.aspx?menuid=189&contentid=54&rptname=bleeding
Factor VII Deficiency Pamphlet—Canadian Hemophilia Society
www.hemophilia.ca/files/engVII.pdf

Support Organizations
National Hemophilia Organization
116 West 32nd Street, 11th Floor
New York, NY 10001
Phone: (212) 328-3700
Fax: (212) 328-3777
Internet: www.hemophilia.org
Hemophilia Federation of America
210 7th Street SE, Suite 200B
Washington, DC 20003
Phone: (800) 230-9797
Fax: (202) 675-6983
Email: info@hemophiliafed.org
Internet: http://hemophiliafed.org

Canadian Hemophilia Society
National Office in Montreal
400-1255 University Street
Montreal, QC H3B 3B6
Phone: (514) 848-0503
Toll free: (800) 668-2686
Fax: (514) 848-9661
Email: chs@hemophilia.ca
Internet: www.hemophilia.ca
The Haemophilia Society
1st Floor, Petersham House
57a Hatton Garden
London, EC1N 8JG
Phone: 020 7831 1020
Free phone helpline: 0800 018 6068
Fax: 020 7405 4824
Email: info@haemophilia.org.uk
Internet: www.haemophilia.org.uk
World Hemophilia Association
1425 René Lévesque Blvd. W., Suite 1010
Montréal, Québec H3G 1T7
Phone: (514) 875-7944
Fax: (514) 875-8916
Email: wfh@wfh.org
Internet: www.whf.org
Aleh Israel Hemophilia Association
PO Box 9013
Ramat Efal 52190
Telefax: 03-9031444
Email: aleh@hemophilia.org.il
Internet: www.hemophilia.org.il

---

1. See section on Glanzmann Thrombasthenia.
2. It is suspected when there is a prolonged prothrombin time (PT) but normal partial thromboplastin time (PTT).
3. At position 244, alanine is replaced by valine, leading to an abnormally functioning protein that is part of factor VII.

4. L. R. Rosenthal, O. Dreskin, and N. Rosenthal, New hemophilia-like disease caused by deficiency of a third plasma thromboplastin factor. Proceeding of the Society of Experimental Biology and Medicine 1953; 82:171–74.

5. U. Seligson, High gene frequency of factor XI (PTA) deficiency in Ashkenazi Jews. *Blood,* 1978; 51:1223–28.

6. Type II mutation causes the amino acid chain to stop prematurely (at the Glu117 location, and thus this mutation is known as Glu117Stop). This results in very low levels of circulating factor XI. People who inherit two copies of the gene with this defect have a mean factor level of 1.2 percent

7. In type III mutation, phenylalanine at the 283 location is replaced by leucine and thus this mutation is also known as Phe283Leu. People who inherit two copies of the gene with this defect have mean factor levels of 9.7 percent. People who inherit one copy of mutation II and one copy of mutation III have mean factor XI levels of 3.3 percent.

8. O. Shpilberg, H. Peretz, A. Zivelin, et al., One of the two common mutations causing factor XI deficiency in Ashkenazi Jews (Type II) is also prevalent in Iraqi Jews, who represent the ancient gene pool of Jews. *Blood,* 1995; 85:429–32.

9. H. Peretz, A. Mulai, S. Usher, et al., The two common mutations causing factor XI deficiency in Jews stem from distinct founders: one of ancient Middle Eastern origin and another of more recent European origin. *Blood,* 1997; 90:2654–59.

Familial Dysautonomia

Summary

Familial dysautonomia is a condition in which the sensory and autonomic nervous systems are inadequately developed. The underdeveloped sensory system leads to lack of sensation and inability to feel pain. The underdevelopment of the autonomic nervous system (which controls involuntary actions) leads to wide swings in blood pressure, excessive sweating, and vomiting. These tend to come in the form of attacks known as *crises*. On an ongoing basis, people with familial dysautonomia tend to have improper functioning of the esophagus, which makes swallowing difficult. This can lead to aspiration and recurrent pneumonia. They also tend to develop severe scoliosis (curvature of the spine) and difficulty walking.

Historical Background

A syndrome that consisted of vomiting and wide swings in blood pressure among five children was first described by Drs. Conrad Riley and Richard Day in 1941. Therefore, this condition is known at times as Riley-Day syndrome. Today the more common nomenclature is familial dysautonomia, a term that reflects the underlying malfunction of the autonomic nervous system and its hereditary nature. This disease is considered one of the hereditary sensory and autonomic neuropathies (HSANs). It is known as HSAN III.

Diagnosis of Condition

Until recently, the diagnosis was clinical. To meet the criteria, the child had to be born to parents of Ashkenazi descent and exhibit the following features: (1) low muscle tone in infancy; (2) decreased or absent tendon reflexes; (3) smooth tongue due to the absence of certain taste buds, leading to decreased ability to taste; (4) absence of tears in response to crying; (5) absence of redness after injection of histamine into the skin; and (6) contraction of the pupil when low doses of a certain medication (methacholine) are placed in the eye. The reaction to these eye drops shows extra sensitivity to this medication, which affects the autonomic nervous system.

In 2001 the gene for this condition was discovered, allowing for direct testing for the disease.

Genetic Cause

The gene associated with familial dysautonomia is the IKBKAP gene found on the long arm of chromosome 9. The mutation in the gene leads to malfunction of the protein produced, called *elongator complex protein 1* (ELP1), particularly in the brain.[1] The main mutation of this gene in those of Ashkenazi Jewish descent is a mutation known as c2204+6T>C.[2]

Heredity

The condition is inherited in an autosomal recessive manner. The carrier frequency among those of Ashkenazi Jewish descent is 1:36. Among those of Polish Ashkenazi Jewish lineage, the carrier frequency is as high as 1:18.

Living with the Condition

The difficulties of hypotonia (low muscle tone), abnormal contractions of the esophagus, and gastrointestinal reflux combine to make proper nutrition challenging. Therefore, it is important to ensure adequate nutrition. This generally involves a combination of thickening feeds for infants and restricting drinking in older children, as well as medication to help with gastrointestinal reflux. In most cases it is recommended that a gastrostomy tube be surgically placed in early childhood to allow for feeding directly into the stomach, and avoiding the risk of foods, especially liquids, entering the lungs. This operation is generally combined with a fundoplication, a procedure that makes the outlet to the esophagus narrower by wrapping part of the stomach around it. The smaller outlet makes it more difficult for the contents of the stomach to be regurgitated and thus reach the lungs.

Repeated pneumonia can lead to chronic lung disease. If this happens, degeneration of the lungs is delayed through treatment methods such as chest physical therapy and antibiotics as needed.

Dry eyes can lead to scarring of the cornea and visual difficulties. People with this condition should use eye lubricants such as artificial tears. They should also have at least annual examinations by an ophthalmologist.

Patients with the condition are at particular risk for kidney disease when they are older. They are also likely to develop curvature of the spine and should be evaluated by an orthopedist. Teeth may be malformed and annual follow-up with a dentist is recommended as well.

Familial dysautonomia used to be associated with death in early childhood, with most children dying before age 10. Now, with improved care that has resulted from the understanding of the condition, the average lifespan has increased to 25 years.

There are two centers in the world that treat this condition. One is located in New York University and headed by Dr. Felicia Axelrod. The other is in Hadassah Hospital in Jerusalem, headed by Dr. Chana Maayan. Through their experience with this condition they have developed a number of recommendations that seem to increase the lifespan. The complete guidelines for care can be obtained via the center at NYU.

Sources
M. Shohat and A. J. Halpern, Familial Dysautonomia. GeneReviews.
http://www.ncbi.nlm.nih.gov/books/NBK1180/

Further Reading
Familial Dysautonomia. Genetics Home Reference.
http://ghr.nlm.nih.gov/condition/familial-dysautonomia/show/print
B. H. Lerner, When diseases disappear—the case of familial dysautonomia. *NEJM* 2009:361:1622–25.

Support Groups
Familial Dysautonomia Foundation
315 West 39th Street, Suite 701
New York, NY 10018
Phone: (212) 279-1066
Internet: www.familialdysautonomia.org
Familial Dysautonomia Hope Foundation (FD Hope)
121 South Estes Drive, Suite 205D
Chapel Hill, NC 27514
Phone: (919) 969-1414
Email: info@fdhope.org
Internet: www.fdhope.org

---

1. Interestingly, those with the mutation are able to produce unaffected ELP1 protein in some other tissues.
2. This is a splice mutation (known as IVS20+6T>C in older nomenclature). The mutation takes place in intron 20. Introns are parts of the DNA that are generally not expressed. However, the shift caused by this mutation leads to improper interpretation of the nearby exons. Rarely (0.5 percent of the time), another mutation called Arg 696Pro (where arginine is replaced by proline in the protein) may be found instead.

Fanconi Anemia

Summary

Fanconi anemia is a multisystem condition that can be caused by a number of genetic mutations. Symptoms can include various congenital malformations, anemia, and bone marrow failure. Patients with this genetic condition are also at a higher risk of developing cancer.

Historical Background

The disease was first described by Guido Fanconi in 1927, when he described three brothers with low levels of all blood components (platelets, white and red blood cells) and other physical abnormalities. In the 1960s it was discovered that the chromosomes of cells cultured from patients with Fanconi anemia were more likely to break when treated with certain chemicals. This finding made it possible to identify patients with the condition even if they did not have other physical abnormalities. It also made it possible to diagnose people with Fanconi anemia who had skeletal abnormalities but no anemia.

Diagnosis of Condition

Some patients are diagnosed soon after birth because of congenital malformations such as absence of thumbs or part of the skeletal system. There can be malformations of other body systems as well. However, the frequency of malformations is quite variable and approximately 25–40 percent of those with the condition have no physical abnormalities.

Others are diagnosed from problems in blood production. The most common situation is progressive bone marrow failure leading to pancytopenia—low levels of all types of blood cells (red blood cells, white blood cells, and platelets)—in childhood. Some will develop aplastic anemia (lack of production of all types of blood cells) as adults. By age 40–48, 90 percent of patients will have developed bone marrow failure. Patients with this condition are at increased risk of developing blood-based cancers such as leukemia (usually acute myelogenous leukemia or AML). Between 10 and 33 percent of those with this condition will have this type of cancer by age 40–48. They are also at increased risk of developing cancer of many solid organs such as the head, neck, or gynecological tract at an unusually young age and in the absence of other risk factors. By age 40–48, the cumulative risk for these kinds of cancers is 28–29 percent.

Genetic Cause

The condition is caused by mutations in a number of different genes. These genes produce proteins that work together to protect the cell from DNA damage. Abnormal proteins decrease the ability of the cell to avoid such damage and thus increase the risk of cancer.

The mutation that is common in those of Ashkenazi Jewish descent occurs within the FANCC gene, located on the long arm of chromosome 9.[1] This gene codes for the Fanconi anemia group C protein.

Heredity

Fanconi anemia is almost always inherited in an autosomal recessive fashion. A child can get it if both parents have a mutation in one of the 13 genes known to be responsible for this condition, even if he or she inherits a different mutation from each parent. Among Ashkenazi Jews, the carrier frequency of the FANCC mutation is approximately 1:90.[2]

If a patient is identified with the condition, it is appropriate to test all siblings, since they may carry the mutation even if they are not yet symptomatic. Because knowing their status makes a difference in their medical care, such as ensuring ongoing monitoring for development of cancer, this genetic screening is clearly needed for the care of the patient and is not subject to halachic debate.

Living with the Condition

Treatment is directed at monitoring for early detection of problems and addressing those that arise. The following are some examples. A complete set of standards for clinical care can be downloaded from the website of the Fanconi Anemia Research Fund (see below).

Regular blood counts (approximately every 3–6 months), supplemented by annual bone marrow biopsies, are performed to monitor the level of all components and allow for early detection of bone marrow failure.

Hormones (androgens) can be given to help delay the onset of bone marrow failure, especially in the production of red blood cells. However, their efficacy tends to wane over time. Medications to boost white cell counts (cytokines) may be tried as well if needed.

If a proper match can be found, stem cell transplantation can cure the problems of bone marrow failure. Successful transplantation will cure the pancytopenia, although the procedure has significant risk. The patient will still be at high risk of developing solid tumors. It is important that the transplant be performed in a center that specializes in Fanconi anemia transplants, since there are modifications that need to be done to the procedure.

Patients need ongoing monitoring for the development of solid tumors and/or leukemia. Monitoring includes annual physical exams, especially of the head and neck, since the risk of tumors in that area is 700 times that of the general public. Any symptoms suggestive of cancer should be evaluated promptly. Women should have an annual pelvic exam including a pap smear. X rays should be avoided as much as possible, because they require radiation that may speed up the process of tumor development.

Orthopedic anomalies may be amenable to surgery. For example, since the thumb is important for the function of the hand, surgery is often performed to create a functional "thumb" from another finger. Occupational therapy may also be of use for learning methods of adaptation.

Nutrition should be monitored; many patients with this condition will have poor nutrition due to gastrointestinal discomfort. While those with the condition tend to be shorter, low weight for height is a sign of malnutrition. Sometimes consultation with a nutritionist and supplemental nutrition will be of help.

Puberty tends to be late in both boys and girls with this condition. Women with Fanconi anemia are fertile, but they tend to undergo early menopause and thus are likely to have a shorter window for childbearing. Men's fertility appears to be unaffected.

Sources
T. Toniguchi. Fanconi Anemia. GeneReviews.
http://www.ncbi.nlm.nih.gov/books/NBK1401/
B. P. Alter and J. M. Lipton, Fanconi Anemia. eMedicine.
http://emedicine/medscape.com/article/960401-overview

Further Reading
Fanconi Anemia. National Heart, Lung and Blood Institute Diseases and Conditions Index. http://www.nhlbi.nih.gov/health/dci/Diseases/fanconi/fanconi_all.html

Support Groups
Fanconi Anemia Research Fund, Inc., and Support Group
1801 Willamette Street, Suite 200
Eugene, OR 97401
Phone: (800) 828-4891 (family support) or (541) 687-4658

Fax: (541) 687-0548
Email: info@fanconi.org
Internet: www.fanconi.org
Fanconi Anemia International Registry
c/o Arleen Auerbach, PhD
Laboratory for Investigative Dermatology
The Rockefeller University
1230 York Avenue
New York, NY 10021-6399
Phone: (212) 327-8862
Canadian Fanconi Anemia Research Fund (Fanconi Canada)
PO Box 38157, Castlewood Postal Outlet
Toronto, ON M5N 3A9
Phone: (416) 489-6393
Fax: (416) 489 6393
Email: admin@fanconicanada.org
Internet: www.fanconicanada.org
European Fanconi Anemia (EUFAR) Center Amsterdam
(A consortium of nine research groups in France, Germany, Italy, United Kingdom, and the Netherlands)
De Boelelaan 1118, 1081 HV
Amsterdam, The Netherlands
Phone: +31 20 - 444 2420
Fax: +31 20 - 444 2422
Email: fanconi.org@VUmc.nl

---

1. The mutation is a splice mutation called IVS4+4A>T (older nomenclature) or c711+4A>T (newer nomenclature). This means that two components of the gene are spliced together, resulting in a single band that is 130 base pairs long instead of two shorter bands of 107 and 103 base pairs each.
2. L. Peleg, R. Pesso, B. Goldman, et al., Bloom syndrome and Fanconi anemia: rate and ethnic origin of mutation carriers in Israel. *IMAJ* 2002; 4:95–97.

Familial Mediterranean Fever

Summary

Familial Mediterranean Fever (FMF) is an inherited disorder consisting of repeated attacks of fever and pain. The pain is due to inflammation of the serous lining (the tissue surrounding the abdominal and chest walls); therefore, this condition is sometimes called *recurrent polyserositis*. Because of the inflammation, patients have attacks of abdominal or chest pain, often accompanied by joint swelling. Some patients with this condition build up a substance known as *amyloid* in the kidneys, which can lead to kidney failure. This complication is most common in Jews of North African origin.

Historical Background

The condition was first described in 1945 by Dr. Sheppard Siegel, an allergist in New York, who described five cases of recurrent attacks of abdominal pain accompanied by high fever. He called the condition *benign paroxysmal peritonitis*, which essentially described the symptoms. The current name, and the discovery that this was a genetic condition inherited in an autosomal recessive manner, is credited to an Israeli team headed by Professor Harry Heller in the early 1960s.

Diagnosis of Condition

Until the end of the 20th century, the diagnosis was only clinical. The disease was suspected when there were recurrent episodes of chest or abdominal pain accompanied by fever. To help give additional evidence that these symptoms represented an attack of FMF, blood tests were done at the time of attacks to look for signs of inflammation, in particular elevated levels of fibrinogen. The diagnosis was often elusive and it was not uncommon for people suffering from the condition to undergo numerous exploratory surgeries before the diagnosis was made. In some patients the symptoms consist of joint swelling and rashes of the legs with fever. These episodes of arthritis and rashes could be confused with many other conditions. Discovery of the underlying genetic mutations has allowed for confirmation of the condition: if these recurrent episodes occur in someone who carries two copies of the mutation, they are probably manifestations of FMF.

When the diagnosis was only clinical, it was thought that this was a condition unique to those of Mediterranean descent. Discovery of the underlying genetic mutation[1] has led to the discovery that many Ashkenazi Jews carry the mutation as well, although manifestations of the disease tend to be rarer and, when they occur, milder.

Genetic Cause

The gene associated with the condition is MEFV, a gene found on the short arm of chromosome 16. The most common mutation of the gene in Jews of North African origin is p.Met694Val.[2] This gene codes for a protein called *pyrin* or *marenostrin*, which is found primarily in white blood cells. It is not completely clear what the purpose of this protein is, but it appears to be associated with modulating inflammation. Therefore, patients with FMF who are lacking this protein have exaggerated episodes of inflammation with the accompanying symptoms of fever and pain in the abdomen and/or chest and possible swelling of the ankles.

Heredity

FMF is inherited in an autosomal recessive manner—both parents have to carry the gene for a person to develop the disease. On the other hand, the severity and frequency of attacks is variable, even within families. The carrier frequency is 1:5 in Jews from Libya and 1:6.5 in Jews from Algeria, Tunisia, and Morocco. In Jews from Iraq and Turkey, the carrier rate is 1:13. Carrier status for at least one mutation has been shown in 1:5 Ashkenazi Jews. However, the disease in Ashkenazi Jews tends to be milder.

Living with the Condition

A major change in the life of patients has been the discovery in 1972 that administration of colchicine can prevent the attacks and, if started early enough in life, can prevent the accumulation of amyloid that causes renal failure. This medication is given as a pill twice daily for life. In those of North African ancestry, this medication is started at a young age and continued through life in order to prevent amyloidosis and renal disease. In Ashkenazi Jews, and Sephardim *not* from North Africa, the purpose is to prevent the attacks. Therefore, decisions about colchicine therapy need to be individualized to the frequency and severity of attacks.

Colchicine can have some side effects. Patients taking the drug need to report to their physicians if they experience muscle pain or weakness, numbness or tingling of fingers or toes, unusual bleeding, or pale lips, tongue, or palms. It is important to note that there are certain medications (such as erythromycin and related antibiotics) and foods (such as grape-fruit juice) that need to be avoided when one is using this medication.

It is recommended that all first-degree relatives of a person diagnosed with the condition, particularly those of North African Jewish descent, should be tested even if asymptomatic. This allows early initiation of colchicine therapy to prevent the accumulation of amyloid and the resultant kidney disease.

Sources
J. O. Meyerhoff, Familial Mediterranean Fever. eMedicine Rheumatology. http://emedicine.medscape.com/article/944157-overview
M. Shohat and G. J. Halpern, Familial Mediterranean Fever. GeneReviews. http://www.ncbi.nlm.nih.gov/books/NBK1227/
E. L. Abel, *Jewish Genetic Disorders*. Jefferson, NC: Macfarland and Co., 2001.
J. Zlotogora, Mendelian Disorders Among Jews. http://www.health.gov.il/Download/pages/bookjews2011.pdf
G. E. Ehrlich, Genetics of Familial Mediterranean Fever and Its Implications. www.annals.org/content/129/7/581

Further Reading
Familial Mediterranean Fever. Genetics Home Reference. http://ghr.nlm.nih.gov/condition/familial-mediterranean-fever
Learning about Familial Mediterranean Fever. National Human Genome Research Institute.
www.genome.gov/pfv.cfm?pageID=12510679

Support Organizations
Anonymous Support Group
http://www.experienceproject.com/groups/Have-Familial-Mediterranean-Fever/95065
Yahoo Group—Familial Mediterranean Fever
http://groups.yahoo.com/group/fmf_support/

---

1. S. Eisenberg, I. Aksentijevich, Z. Deng, D. L. Kastner, and Y. Matzner, Diagnosis of familial Mediterranean fever by a molecular genetics method. *Ann Intern Med* 1998; 129:539–42.
2. Valine replaces methionine at position 694 of the protein, leading to a less active form of the protein, which is less able to control the process of inflammation.

Gaucher Disease

Summary

Gaucher disease is a condition caused by lack of the enzyme *glucosylceramidase*. It is characterized by bone disease, enlarged liver and/or spleen, and anemia. There may be lung disease as well. Symptoms can range from very mild to severe.

There are several different forms of Gaucher disease. The form that is predominant in people of Ashkenazi Jewish descent is Type 1. Unlike other forms of Gaucher disease, Type 1 does not affect the central nervous system.

Historical Background

A woman with an enlarged liver and spleen was described by Dr. Philippe Gaucher in 1882.

Diagnosis of Condition

The diagnosis is suspected in cases of bone disease (often first seen as an incidental finding on an X-ray), enlarged liver or spleen, or unexplained anemia. The confirmatory test is a measure of the level of glucosylceramidase enzyme activity in white blood cells or other cells with nuclei. An activity level less than 15 percent of normal indicates the disease.

Carriers usually have an activity level that is half of normal. However, there is so much overlap between the level of carriers and normal levels that activity level cannot be used to screen for carriers. When a family history of the disease is known, then testing can be done for the genetic mutation found in that family.

Genetic Cause

The gene associated with Gaucher disease, known as GBA, is found on the long arm of chromosome 1. Many of the mutations of this gene lead to reduced production of an enzyme known as *acid beta-cosylceramidase* (also called *glucosylceramidase* and *glucocerebrosidase*). In those of Ashkenazi Jewish descent, the disease is caused, almost 90 percent of the time, by one of four mutations. Screening for six mutations (N370S, 84GG, L444P, IVS2+1G>a,V394L, R496H)[1] can detect 90–95 percent of all carriers.

The affected enzyme is needed for the breakdown of *glucocerebroside*. This is a *glycolipid* (form of fat molecule to which a sugar molecule is attached) that results from the breakdown of blood cells, especially white blood cells. The extra glucocerebroside that is not broken down builds up in the macrophage cells of the bones, liver, and spleen, whose job is to "eat up" old and dying cells. A cell that is stuffed with the lipid that cannot be broken down has a specific appearance under the microscope (as if crumpled up tissue paper was pushing the nucleus of the cell to the side) and is known as a *Gaucher cell*.

The build-up of Gaucher cells in the bones can lead to weak bones (*osteopenia*) and fractures from little or no trauma. It can also cut off the blood supply in the bone, leading to infarction (death of cells), which can cause severe bone pain known as *painful crises*. The build-up in the cells of the liver and spleen is what makes them large. The replacement of the blood-producing elements of the bone marrow with Gaucher cells, coupled with the increased removal of blood cells by an enlarged spleen, are what cause the anemia (lack of red blood cells that carry oxygen) and *thrombocytopenia* (lack of platelets needed for clotting) associated with this condition.

Heredity

Gaucher disease is an autosomal recessive disease. A person who inherits a mutation from each parent, even if not the same mutation, will be affected. Those who inherit two copies of the N370S mutation tend to have a later onset and relatively mild course. Carriers of the disease are not at risk of getting the disorder, but, because the symptoms of the disease can be mild, it is possible for an adult to have the condition without being aware of it.

The frequency of carrying any mutation of the GBA gene in those of Ashkenazi Jewish descent is estimated at one in 15 people.

Living with the Condition

Presentation of the disease in those with two copies of an affected gene can be quite varied. Some will suffer painful crises from a young age, some will have mild anemia and enlarged livers and/or spleens, and others will be unaffected until very late in life if at all.

There are several forms of treatment for Gaucher disease. They include relief of specific symptoms, enzyme replacement therapy, and substrate reduction therapy.

In symptomatic treatment, pain crises are handled with pain relief and hydration. Transfusion of blood may be needed for severe anemia.

Splenectomy (removal of the spleen) is done to help deal with the pressure of the spleen on other organs and to improve the anemia. Calcium, vitamin D, and oral bisphosphonates may be taken to alleviate low bone density. Joint replacement may be needed in some cases where there has been joint destruction. Care is best handled with the assistance of Comprehensive Gaucher Centers.

Many of these treatments are no longer needed today because of the availability of enzyme replacement therapy. The most commonly used enzyme replacement at present, produced in hamster ovary cells by recombinant DNA, is called *imiglucerase* (brand name Cerezyme). This replaces an older form of enzyme, marketed as Ceredase, that was obtained from human placentas. A new recombinant enzyme produced in cultured human cells, called *velaglucerase alfa* (VPRIV), has recently been approved. Decisions about whether, when, and how to use enzyme replacement therapy need to be made with the guidance of a specialist (generally either geneticist or hematologist). The therapy is particularly helpful for the symptoms of anemia and the enlarged organs. Treatment of the pain crises may still be needed since the bone manifestations take the longest time to respond. These treatments are given intravenously.

Another approach to treating symptomatic patients who cannot use enzyme replacement therapy is substrate reduction therapy. In this approach, instead of replacing the missing enzyme, the substance on which the enzyme works is reduced. The current medication is *miglustat* (brand name Zavesca), which inhibits the enzyme glucosylceramide synthatase and thus reduces the production of glucosylceramide, the substrate of the missing enzyme. This drug is given orally.

Consensus guidelines for monitoring this condition include a history and physical exam every 6–12 months, monitoring of anemia via a complete blood count, and monitoring liver function enzymes and clotting factors and growth. Bone X-rays can help detect changes due to Gaucher disease as well as help monitor skeletal maturity. Dual energy X-ray absorptiometry (DEXA) can be used to detect and follow bone density. A chest X-ray can help determine if there is pulmonary involvement.

Sources

E. Sidransky, Gaucher Disease. eMedicine.
http://emedicine.medscape.com/article/944157-overview
G. M. Pastores and D. A. Hughes, Gaucher Disease. GeneReviews.
http://www.ncbi.nlm.nih.gov/books/NBK1269/

E. L. Abel, *Jewish Genetic Disorders*. Jefferson, NC: Macfarland and Co., 2001.

Further Reading
MedicineNet.com. Gaucher Disease.
http://www.medicinenet.com/gaucher_disease/article.htm
Gaucher Disease. Genetics Home Reference.
http://ghr.nlm.nih.gov/condition/gaucher-disease

Support Organizations
National Gaucher Foundation
2227 Idelwood Road, Suite G
Tucker, GA 30084
Phone: (800) 504-3189
Fax: (779) 934-2911
Email: ngf@gaucherdisease.org
Internet: www.gaucherdisease.org
Gaucher Association
3 Bull Pitch
Dursley, Gloucestershire GL11 4NG
Phone/Fax: +44 1453 549 231
Internet: www.gaucher.org.uk
National Gaucher Foundation of Canada
4100 Yonge Street, Suite 610
North York, ON M2P 285
Phone: (613) 521-5050
Email: christinewhite@gauchercanada.ca
Internet: www.gauchercanada.ca

---

1. The four mutations in the panel are N370S, 84GG, L444P, and IVS2+1. The additional two mutations are V394L and R496H.

N370S is a point mutation where adenine is replaced by cytosine in the DNA at position 1226. As a result, asparagine is replaced by serine in position 409 (or 370) of the protein.

84GG (also called c85insG or c93_94insG) is a frame shift mutation where guanine is inserted. The position number of the insertion varies with the counting system, which is why there are multiple names. The result of this mutation is that alanine replaces leucine in position 29 of the protein.

L444P, in codon 1448 of the DNA, is a mutation where thymine is replaced by cytosine. As a result, the protein will have proline in place of leucine.

IVS2+ (or IVS2+1G>A) is a splice mutation where two parts of the sequence are combined, leading to an abnormal protein.

V394L is a point mutation where thymine replaces guanine at position 1297. This leads to leucine replacing valine at position 433 (or 394 depending on nomenclature) of the protein.

R496H is a point mutation where adenine replaces guanine in position 1604 of the DNA, leading to the replacement of arginine by histidine at position 535 of the protein.

Glanzmann Thrombasthenia

Summary

Glanzmann thrombasthenia is a condition in which the platelets lack a receptor that allows them to aggregate (clump together) to stop bleeding at sites of injury to a blood vessel.[1] The number of platelets and their appearance under the microscope is normal; however, the platelets cannot gather together in a normal manner to allow for coagulation. The most common bleeding symptoms are nosebleed, bruising, and bleeding from gums. Women with this condition have long and heavy periods.

The severity of the condition is quite variable. It can range from minimal bruising to severe hemorrhage. There is no clear correlation between the amount of functional receptor remaining and the severity of bleeding complications.

Historical Background

The condition was described by Dr. Eduard Glanzmann, a Swiss pediatrician, in 1918.

Diagnosis of Condition

The condition is suspected in those of Iraqi origin when there is bruising or prolonged bleeding. It may first appear in newborns or at a later age after a tooth extraction. Tests of platelet function are done to rule out other causes of platelet malfunction or clotting disorders. In those of Iraqi Jewish origin, tests for the specific mutation can be performed.

Genetic Cause

Each part of the receptor is coded for by a different gene. The gene that is most commonly affected in the Iraqi Jewish populations is the GPII-Ia gene located on chromosome 17.[2]

Heredity

This condition is inherited in an autosomal recessive manner. Carriers of the condition are generally asymptomatic, although they have a reduced level of the receptor (approximately 60 percent of normal). The carrier frequency in the Iraqi Jewish population is approximately 1:115.

Living with the Condition

Individuals with this condition need to avoid using medications that can further interfere with clotting. These include aspirin, nonsteroidal anti-inflammatory drugs (NSAIDS) such as ibuprofen, and heparin and warfarin.

To prevent bleeding disorders, a medication known as *desmopressin* (DDAVP) may be used. When there is a bleeding episode, or prior to surgery, individuals often need platelet transfusions. Use of recombinant Factor VIIa may help reduce the need for transfusions.

Frequent need for platelet transfusion raises the risk of acquiring blood-borne diseases. Therefore, immunization against Hepatitis B is particularly important. Special care needs to be taken when platelet transfusions are given, to reduce the chance of patients developing antibodies against platelets.

Bleeding from the gums is more likely when there is poor dental hygiene. Therefore, attention to good dental hygiene is particularly important in those with this condition.

Bleeding with menses can be difficult to manage. For women who are not trying to become pregnant, extended use of hormonal contraception can minimize both the frequency of menses and the degree of bleeding. Childbirth needs to be managed in conjunction with a hematologist familiar with this condition.

Sources

Z. Ashraf and M. J. Shumate, Glanzmann Thrombasthenia. eMedicine Hematology.
http://emedicine.medscape.com/article/200311-overview
A. T. Nurden, Glanzmann thrombasthenia, *Orphanet Encyclopedia*, September 2005.
www.orpha.net/data/patho/GB/uk-Glanzmann.pdf
E. L. Abel, *Jewish Genetic Disorders*. Jefferson, NC: Macfarland and Co., 2001.

Further Reading

Glanzmann's Disease. *MedlinePlus Encyclopedia*
http://www.nlm.nih.gov/medlineplus/ency/article/001305.htm

Support Organizations
Glanzmann's Research Foundation
Phone: (706) 533-4818
Internet: www.glanzmanns.com
Glanzmann's Thrombasthenia Contact Group
28 Duke Road
Newton, Hyde SK14 4JB
Phone: 0161 368 0219
Email: mbuxton5505@yahoo.co.uk

----

1. The missing receptor is a complex of two subunits known as IIb and IIIa, or in more modern nomenclature αIIb and β3. A defect in either of them means that the complex will not function.
2. The most common mutation in this population (over 85 percent) is an 11-base pair deletion within exon 12. This gene codes for the beta portion of the complex. An abnormal beta portion of the complex leads to the clotting difficulties found in this condition.

Glucose-6-Phosphate Dehydrogenase (G6PD) Deficiency

Melissa Meyers

Summary

G6PD deficiency is a condition in which the enzyme *glucose-6-dehydrogenase* is missing in blood cells. This enzyme is involved in the production of *NADPH*, a substance that helps protect red blood cells against bursting apart from exposure to oxygen in the body. If individuals with this deficiency are exposed to certain foods or medications, or develop an infection, the blood cells may burst apart—a process called *hemolysis*.

Hemolytic anemia associated with G6PD deficiency can present with a variety of symptoms, including back and abdominal pain, jaundice, enlarged spleen, and a yellowing of the eyes called *scleral icterus*. Abdominal pain typically increases four to seven days after hemolysis. Occasionally, a bout of hemolytic anemia may warrant a blood transfusion. All G6PD-deficient individuals are at increased risk for developing *sepsis*, a dangerous form of blood-borne infection, and other sepsis-related complications after a severe injury. Repeated bouts of hemolytic anemia can lead to the production of gallstones.

G6PD deficiency is an extremely common condition, affecting approximately 400 million people worldwide. It is postulated that the reason it is so prevalent, especially in those parts of the world where malaria is (or was) rampant, is that being heterozygous for the condition provides some degree of protection against malaria.

Historical Background

In 1953, Dr. Ernest Beutler identified the enzyme deficiency among a population of patients suffering from severe anemia after receiving the drug primaquine as a treatment for malaria. Beutler went on to develop the first tests to identify the disease.

Diagnosis of Condition

The disease is suspected and often tested for at birth in those areas of the world with a high incidence of the condition, such as the Middle East. It can sometimes present in infancy as prolonged jaundice. It is also suspected when a patient has an episode of hemolytic anemia, especially if he or she is of an ethnic background where the condition is common. The condition is confirmed by a fluorescent spot test, also known as a *quantitative spectrophotometric* analysis.

Genetic Cause

The G6PD gene is found on the long arm of the X chromosome. There are over 300 reported mutations to date. These varied mutations can produce a number of variants. The most common variant among Sephardi Jews of Kurdish, Iranian, Iraqi, and Italian descent is the Mediterranean variant.

Heredity

Most variants of the disease, including the Mediterranean variant, are found on the distal long arm of the X chromosome. Because of this, males are most often affected, since they have only one X chromosome, whereas females have two X chromosomes, one of which is generally still healthy. G6PD deficiency has been reported in heterozygous women, who carry one affected and one normal copy of the chromosome. However, the condition is generally milder. A heterozygous woman can pass this condition on to her sons, even if she is not affected.

Carrier frequency of the Mediterranean variant in Iranian and Iraqi Jewish populations has been reported in up to 1:4 males, and in 1:27 among those from Yemen.

Living with the Condition

Individuals with G6PD may undergo hemolysis with certain triggers. Therefore, the main goal is to avoid such triggers. Common perpetrators of hemolytic attacks include antimalarial drugs (primaquine, chloraquine, pamaquine, pentaquine) and several antibiotics (most sulfa drugs, nitrofurantoin, naladixic acid, chloremphenicol). Eating fava beans can also trigger attacks in those with the Mediterranean variant. It is important to avoid exposure to certain other chemicals such as mothballs (naphthalene). Nursing mothers of G6PD-deficient infants should be careful to avoid those medications that can cause hemolysis, since they may be passed to the baby through breast milk. Certain infections can also lead to a hemolytic reaction and should be treated by a physician familiar with hemolytic anemias. Since the disease affects mostly very young and very old blood cells, continued infection or ingestion of an oxidative trigger typically does not cause prolonged symptoms.

Sources
S. M. Carter and S. J. Gross, Glucose-6-Phosphate Dehydrogenase Deficiency. eMedicine Hematology.
http://emedicine.medscape.com/article/200390-overview
J. D. Frank, Diagnosis and Management of G6PD Deficiency. *Am Fam Physician*. 2005; 72:1277–82.
J. Zlotogara, Mendelian Disorders Among Jews. www.health.gov.il/Download/pages/book_jews7.pdf

Further Reading
Glucose-6-phosphate Dehydrogenase Deficiency. Genetics Home Reference.
http://ghr.nlm.nih.gov/condition/glucose-6-phosphate-dehydrogenase-deficiency. Accessed July 2, 2010.
Sephardic Jewish Genetic Diseases Resource. http://www.victorcenters.org/sephardi-info.cfm.

Support Organizations
G6PD Organization
Internet: www.g6pd.org

Glycogen Storage Diseases

Summary

Glycogen storage diseases occur when the liver lacks the ability to break down glycogen, a substance that the body uses to store glucose. Glycogen is found primarily in the liver, and also in the muscles. A number of different enzymes are needed to release the glucose from the glycogen for use as a quick source of energy.

In glycogen storage diseases, the build-up of glycogen leads to an enlarged liver. Because the liver cannot release glucose to maintain a steady level of blood glucose between meals, affected people have episodes of *hypoglycemia* (low blood sugar). This can be exacerbated by illnesses that cause vomiting or prevent frequent eating. Inability to release the nutrition from glucose also leads to poor growth and delayed development of puberty in many children.

There are seven different glycogen storage diseases known to date. Different enzymes are affected in each type. Defects in two of these enzymes are associated with Jewish lineage.

Type I

Glycogen storage disease (GSD) type 1, also known as *Von Gierke disease* for the physician who first described the condition, happens when the liver cells cannot break down glycogen because of the lack of the enzyme *glucose 6 phosphatase* (G6Pase). In addition to the symptoms described above, abnormal biochemical pathways caused by this genetic defect lead to the build-up of lactic acid and uric acid. The extra lactic acid can turn the blood acidic (*lactic acidosis*) and lead to a feeling of fatigue. Elevated levels of uric acid can lead to the formation of kidney stones.

Before management of the condition was understood, it was generally fatal in early childhood. Currently, dietary management has allowed people to live into adulthood. At older ages, problems with kidney function as well as liver tumors can develop. People affected with this condition are generally short. They also tend to be prone to bleeding due to the platelet dysfunction that accompanies this condition. Although they have high levels of cholesterol, they are rarely affected by hardening of the arteries.

Historical Background

An association between enlarged livers and disturbed glycogen metabolism was first reported in 1929 by Edgar Otto Conrad Von Gierke, a

German pathologist, based on autopsy of two children whose livers and kidneys were enlarged and contained excessive glycogen. In 1952 Drs. Carl and Gerty Cori, a husband and wife team, discovered that the condition was due to deficiency of G6Pase. The link to chromosome 17 was reported in 1993.

Diagnosis of Condition

The condition may be suspected immediately after birth if there is neonatal hypoglycemia that is not explained by other risk factors such as a diabetic mother. The condition is also suspected in infants (generally aged 3–4 months) with enlarged livers combined with symptoms of hypoglycemia such as fussiness, lethargy, or seizures. There are generally elevated levels of lactic acid, uric acid, and lipids. The affected children also often have pudgy cheeks that give them a "doll-like" appearance. The condition can be confirmed when decreased levels of enzyme are found in cells obtained by liver biopsy. If a specific mutation is known in the family or is suspected on the basis of ethnic origin, genetic mutational analysis may confirm the diagnosis without the need for liver biopsy.

Genetic Cause

A mutation in the gene for glucose-6-phosphatase (G6Pase), found on chromosome 17, causes a deficiency of this enzyme. Without this enzyme, the body cannot release the glucose that is stored in the liver as glycogen. This means that without frequent eating, those with this condition will develop low blood sugar and its associated symptoms of dizziness, seizure, and coma. The build-up also causes enlargement of the liver, which can be found on physical examination.

Deficiency of G6Pase is known as GSD Type Ia. Deficiency of another enzyme (*glucose-6-phosphate translocase*, or G6PT), causes GSD Type Ib. Type Ia is more common among Ashkenazi Jews. The mutation leading to the deficiency in this population is R83C.[1]

Heredity

The condition is inherited in an autosomal recessive manner. The carrier frequency for this mutation in the Ashkenazi Jewish population is 1:71. Prevalence of GSD Type Ia is five times more common in those of Ashkenazi Jewish descent than in the general Caucasian population.

Living with the Condition

The key to preventing the episodes of hypoglycemia is to provide ongoing access to glucose. This is accomplished in young children through frequent feeding and through feeding glucose by tube to the stomach (either via the nose or via surgical insertion through the abdomen). In older children and adults, eating uncooked cornstarch provides a source of glucose that is broken down slowly. Other sugars such as lactose, sucrose, and fructose need to be limited.

Home blood glucose monitoring can help ensure adequate glucose provision. Home blood ketone monitoring can help ensure good control, as high levels of ketones mean that the body is breaking down fat instead of using glucose as a source of energy—a sign that not enough glucose is available.

Nutritional supervision with monitoring of growth and development is important to make sure that proper nutrition is provided. Iron supplements and vitamin D may be necessary. Careful compliance with the regimen can lead to normal growth and puberty. Lifetime compliance is challenging to the affected person and his family. Psychosocial support should be considered in helping the family deal with the situation.

High levels of cholesterol or uric acid, if present, are treated as needed. Starting in adolescence, the kidneys and the liver are generally monitored by ultrasound for the development of stones and size, respectively. Special preparation is needed before surgery to prevent bleeding complications.

Individuals with this condition should not fast, even on Yom Kippur. If they become ill and are not willing to eat, they need hospitalization to provide intravenous glucose.

Sources

D. S. Bali and Y. T. Chen, Glycogen Storage Disease Type I. GeneReviews. http://www.ncbi.nlm.nih.gov/books/NBK1312/

K. S. Roth, Glycogen Storage Disease Type I. eMedicine Pediatrics. http://emedicine.medscape.com/article/949937-overview

H. Ozen, Glycogen storage diseases: new perspectives. *World J Gastroenterol* 2007; 13:2541–53.

Further Reading

Type 1 Glycogen Storage Disease. Association for Glycogen Storage Disease
www.agsdus.org/html/typeiprintable.html

Type III
Summary

Glycogen storage disease (GSD) Type III occurs when the liver and muscle cells cannot break down glycogen because of the lack of the enzyme *amylo-1,6-glucosidase* (AGD), also known as *debranching enzyme* (GDE).

In the form of GSD Type III known as IIIa, the AGD enzyme is missing in the muscle cells as well, and *dextrin*, a breakdown product of glycogen, builds up in these cells. Therefore, people with this condition tend to develop progressive muscle weakness. For this reason, GSDIIIa is also considered a muscular dystrophy—a muscle weakness disease. Dextrin can accumulate in the muscle tissue of the heart as well.

The episodes of hypoglycemia are most common in the first decade of life and in some people can resolve with puberty. However, liver disease, including liver failure and liver cancer, can occur later in life. The muscle weakness that develops over time can range from mild to severe.

Historical Background

The first description of two patients with the symptoms of this condition was published in 1938 by Drs. I. Snappes and Simon van Creveld. In 1953 Dr. Gilbert Burnett Forbes described a third patient and suggested that the substance that had built up in the liver and the muscle of this patient had an abnormal structure. Drs. B. Illingworth and Gerty Cori identified this substance to be a breakdown product of glycogen that Drs. Carl and Gerty Cori had previously called a *limit dextrin.* For this reason, the condition is also called limit dextrinosis, Cori disease, Forbes disease, or Cori-Forbes disease.

Diagnosis of Condition

The condition is suspected when there are episodes of hypoglycemia. These tend to start around 3–4 months of age when feeding frequency decreases, rather than during the newborn period. The condition may also be suspected when an enlarged liver is found on physical exam, or it may be suspected in an older child with progressive muscle weakness. Diagnosis is confirmed at present by the finding of reduced levels of the AGD enzyme in liver cells, obtained by biopsy. Outside the United States, initial screening may be done by testing for the level of AGD in white blood cells. Muscle involvement is ascertained by muscle biopsy. Genetic mutational analysis of the AGL gene may confirm the diagnosis without the need for liver biopsy. This is especially true in certain ethnic groups such as those of North African Jewish descent.

Genetic Cause

A mutation in the AGL gene for the glycogen debranching enzyme, found on the short arm of chromosome 1, causes a deficiency of this enzyme. Lack of the enzyme means that glycogen is only partially broken down—the main backbone of the molecule, which is broken down by a different enzyme, can be cleaved, but the branches of the molecule are still intact. Therefore, only some of the glucose stored in the glycogen can be released, and without frequent eating, those with this condition can develop low blood sugar and its associated symptoms of dizziness, irritability, and even seizures and coma. The dextrin build-up in the liver leads to an enlarged liver that can be found on physical examination, and sometimes to liver dysfunction. Build-up in the heart muscle can lead to heart dysfunction. Build-up in the muscle cells leads to progressive muscle weakness.

The condition is more common in Jews of North African origin, especially from Morocco. The type of disease in this population is IIIa. The mutation leading to the deficiency in this population is 4455delT.[2]

Heredity

The condition is inherited in an autosomal recessive manner. The carrier rate among Jews of North African origin is estimated to be 1:37.

Living with the Condition

The key to preventing the episodes of hypoglycemia is to provide ongoing access to glucose. This is done in young children by frequent feeding and giving glucose by tube feeding at night. It is important that the feeding apparatus be attached to a pump with an alarm to ensure that the infusion does not accidentally stop at night, which can lead to dangerous hypoglycemia. In older children and adults, eating uncooked cornstarch provides a source of glucose that is broken down slowly. As in Type I, home monitoring is available to help maintain proper glucose levels.

Nutritional supervision with monitoring of growth and development is needed to make sure that proper nutrition is provided. Sugars such as fructose do not need to be avoided, but overall sugar intake should be moderate. Many recommend a higher protein diet to keep the body from using the amino acids of the muscle proteins as a source of fuel. As with GSD I, fasting should be avoided.

It is important to monitor heart function of those with this condition. Current recommendations are for yearly echocardiograms and electrocardiograms every other year. If an abnormality is found, care should be managed individually by a cardiologist.

Follow-up of liver function with blood tests is important. It is expected that the liver function tests will be elevated, but ongoing monitoring will identify deterioration of function and assist in deciding whether a liver transplant is needed. Care should be taken to avoid medications and substances such as alcohol, which can damage the liver. Special attention should be given to vaccinating against hepatitis A and B.

Evaluation of strength and development should be ongoing, since muscle weakness can be subtle. Physical therapy can help maximize function. Assistance in getting adaptive equipment, if needed, may be possible through the Muscular Dystrophy Association.

Individuals with this condition can have elevated levels of cholesterol and lipids. Use of statins, a type of medication used for elevated cholesterol, is not recommended, because it can exacerbate the muscle weakness.

Women with this condition should avoid hormonal contraception (estrogen in particular) because of their already increased risk of liver adenomas (benign tumors). Pregnant women with this condition need additional monitoring because their glucose needs will increase. In the last trimester, it is especially important to maintain ketone levels in the normal range since elevated ketones can lead to preterm labor.

Sources
A. Dagli, C. P. Sentner, and D. A. Weinstein, Glycogen Storage Disease Type III. GeneReviews.
http://www.ncbi.nlm.nih.gov/books/NBK26372/
W. E. Anderson, Glycogen Storage Disease Type III. eMedicine Endocrinology.
http://emedicine.medscape.com/article/119597-overview
D. H. Tegay and R. Jose, Glycogen Storage Disease Type III. eMedicine Pediatrics.
http://emedicine.medscape.com/article/942618-overview
P. S. Kishnani, S. L. Austin, P. Arn, et al., Glycogen Storage Disease Type III diagnosis and management guidelines. *Genetics in Medicine* 2010;12:446–463.

Further Reading
Type III Glycogen Storage Disease. Association for Glycogen Storage Disease
http://www.agsdus.org/html/typeiiicori.htm

Support Organizations
Association for Glycogen Storage Disease
PO Box 896
Durant, IA 52747
Phone: (563) 514-4022
Internet: www.agsdus.org
Association for Glycogen Storage Disease (UK)
9 Lindop Road
Hale, Altrincham, Cheshire, WA15 9DZ
Internet: www.agsd.org.uk
The Children's Fund for Glycogen Storage Disease Research
Wendy and David Feldman
917 Bethany Mountain Road
Chesire, CT 06410
Phone: (203) 272-CURE (2873)
Email: info@curegsd.org
Internet: www.curegsd.org
Muscular Dystrophy Association—USA
National Headquarters
3300 East Sunrise Drive
Tucson, AZ 85718
Phone: (800) 572-1717
Email: mda@mdausa.org
Internet: www.mda.org

---

1. This is a point mutation where arginine is replaced by cysteine at position 83. Therefore, it is also written at times as pArg83Cys.
2. A deletion of threonine at position 4455. This leads to production of a truncated enzyme that does not function.

Hyperinsulinism of Infancy

Summary

Hyperinsulinism of infancy (HI) is a condition in which the beta cells of the pancreas produce too much insulin. If people with this disorder are not fed frequently enough, the high levels of insulin lead to episodes of hypoglycemia (low blood sugar), which can cause seizures and brain damage.

There are a number of forms of the condition. The form that is more common in those of Ashkenazi Jewish origin is *diffuse hyperinsulinemia* (diffuse HI), where all the beta cells of the pancreas are affected. This form is also known as *persistent hyperinsulinemic hypoglycemia of infancy* (PHHI), *congenital hyperinsulinism*, *familial hyperinsulinism,* or *nesidioblastosis* (which is derived from the Greek words for islet germ cell tumor).

Historical Background

Hypoglycemia in newborns is well known. A severe form of it was described at the beginning of the 20th century and was called *nesidioblastosis*, a term that describes the abnormal microscopic appearance of the pancreas of some of those who died with this condition. Since the 1980s, the preferred term is *hyperinsulinism of infancy* (HI).

The genetic basis for hyperinsulinism of infancy has been elucidated over the last few decades. The increased incidence in Ashkenazi Jews has been noted, as well as the specific genetic defect that is more common.

Diagnosis of Condition

The severe neonatal form of this disease is suspected when a newborn has unexpected hypoglycemia. The symptoms of hypoglycemia are jitteriness, poor feeding, and/or seizures. What differentiates congenital hyperinsulinism from the more common hypoglycemia, which can occur in newborns born to diabetic mothers or who are overly stressed surrounding birth, is that it does not resolve with treatment of the underlying condition (such as warming the baby, treating an infection, or temporarily providing glucose).

At times, the disease is less severe and appears first in childhood. In that case, it is suspected when there are repeated episodes of hypoglycemia, generally of a milder nature. Since the onset is less dramatic, the later onset form is generally harder to recognize.

The condition is confirmed by measuring levels of insulin, which are found to be elevated. Additional blood and urine tests may be done to rule out other causes of the low blood sugar. Since the levels of insulin can greatly fluctuate in mild cases, it can be more difficult to reach a definite diagnosis in such cases.

When a specific genetic mutation is known to exist in a family, or is suspected based on ethnic origin such as Ashkenazi Jewish background, this mutation can be tested for.

Genetic Cause

HI can be caused by mutations in five different genes on chromosome 11. Diffuse HI is most often caused by a defect in the gene known as ABCC8.[1, 2] In those of Ashkenazi Jewish descent, two specific mutations (pPhe 1387 del,[3] and c3989-9g>a[4]) account for more than 90 percent of all cases.

Heredity

The form of HI that is more common in those of Ashkenazi Jewish descent is inherited in an autosomal recessive manner. Both parents have to be carriers of the gene. However, especially in those cases that have the splice mutation (c3989-9g>a), the severity of the condition can vary between family members, even to the point where some homozygous individuals are asymptomatic. The carrier frequency in the Ashkenazi Jewish population has not yet been determined.

Living with the Condition

Initial treatment of the condition is medical. Effort is made to ensure constant access to glucose through frequent feeding. With newborns, a naso-gastric (NG) tube is generally placed to ensure constant feeding, especially overnight. If tube feeding is continued for a long time, this NG tube is generally replaced by a tube surgically inserted through the abdominal wall directly into the stomach (G tube). A number of medications (such as diazoxide, chlorothiazide, octeotide, nifedipine) are generally tried to determine whether one drug or a combination of drugs can reduce the insulin secretion and prevent hypoglycemia.

Blood glucose levels need to be monitored frequently throughout the day. For older children, parents generally need to keep sugared drinks and snacks on hand at all times to give in case of hypoglycemia. They should also have ready access to glucagon. Injection of glucagon can raise blood sugar for approximately one hour in emergency cases when the person cannot eat.

If medical stabilization works, that is sufficient treatment. After a period of time ranging from months to years, control of glucose tends to get easier. However, many infants reach a point where it is too difficult to manage the situation medically and undergo surgery to remove the greater part of their pancreas. The markedly reduced amount of beta cells that are left are then insufficient to produce hypoglycemia and the child can be fed normally. However, over time, this reduced amount of beta cells becomes insufficient to produce enough insulin and the child will develop diabetes and need to be treated with insulin.

Sources
R. S. Gillespie and S. Ponder, Persistent Hyperinsulinemic Hypoglycemia of Infancy. eMedicine Pediatrics.
http://emedicine.medscape.com/article/923538-overview
B. Glaser, Familial Hyperinsulinism (FHI). GeneReviews.
http://www.ncbi.nlm.nih.gov/books/NBK1375/
E. L. Abel, *Jewish Genetic Disorders*. Jefferson, NC: Macfarland and Co., 2001.

Further Reading
Familial Hyperinsulinism. Genetics Home Reference.
http://ghr.nlm.nih.gov/condition/familial-hyperinsulinism

Support Organizations
Congenital Hyperinsulinemia International
5 Sierra Blanca Road
Cedar Crest, NM 87008
Email: MHopkins@CongenitalHI.org
Internet: www.congenitalhi.org
Congenital Hyperinsulinism Center
Children's Hospital of Philadelphia
34th Street and Civic Center Boulevard
Philadelphia, PA 19104
Phone: (215) 590-7682
Internet: www.chop.edu/service/congenital-hyperinsulinism-center

Children's Hyperinsulinism Fund
c/o Clare Gilbert
MEGGA DSN Office
Level 10, Southwood Building
Great Ormond Street Hospital for Children NHS Trust
London WC1N3JH
Phone: 020 74059200, ext. 0360
Email: info@hi-fund
Internet: www.hi-fund.org
Website for Families of Children with Hyperinsulinism
www.sur1.org
Yahoo Group—Hyperinsulinism
http://health.groups.yahoo.com/group/hyperins
Yahoo Group—Hyperinsulinism for children and teenagers
http://health.groups.yahoo.com/group/hyperinsulinism_kids

---

1. This gene used to be called SUR1.
2. Defects in this gene lead to production of defective channels (known as KATP, for ATP-dependent potassium channels) in the beta cells of the pancreas, which then produce too much insulin.
3. A deletion of phenylalanine at position 1387. Due to differences in how the positions are counted, this is called at times pPhe1388.
4. This is a splice mutation, where two parts of the gene not usually in sequence are brought together.

Joubert Syndrome

Summary

Joubert syndrome is the constellation of symptoms that results from lack of proper development of the *cerebellar vermis*, the area of the brain that controls coordination and balance. The symptoms include breathing too fast (hyperpnea), low muscle tone (hypotonia), inability to control voluntary movements (ataxia), and jerky eye movements (ocular apraxia). Mental development is delayed as well. Some cases are associated with degeneration of the kidneys or the retina. Some are associated with extra fingers or toes.

Many cases of this condition are sporadic, meaning that they occur without a family history. Some cases, however, are familial. Recently, a specific genetic mutation has been found to be associated with this condition in families of Ashkenazi Jewish descent.

Historical Background

In 1969 Marie Joubert, a Canadian neurologist, described the condition in four siblings whose parents were related to each other. In 1977 the condition was given Dr. Joubert's name.

Diagnosis of Condition

The condition is suspected when the clinical features described above are present. An MRI (magnetic resonance imaging) of the brain will confirm the underlying structural abnormality. The typical finding on MRI is known as the *molar tooth sign*. The underdevelopment of the cerebellar vermis causes other parts of the cerebellum to be elongated and very much resembles a molar tooth. To fit the diagnosis of classic Joubert syndrome, this sign needs to be present. There are other conditions that overlap the classic description of Joubert syndrome; these are known as *Joubert syndrome and related disorders*. It is not yet clear if these are separate entities or subtypes of Joubert syndrome.

In the general population, four genes have been associated with Joubert syndrome. However, only 10 percent of cases are associated with one of these four mutations. In those of Ashkenazi Jewish descent, all the cases tested to date have been associated with a particular mutation.

Genetic Cause

Mutations of a number of genes have been linked to this condition. In 2010, through testing requested by Dor Yesharim,[1] an association was found between a mutation in the TMEM216 gene on chromosome 11 and Joubert syndrome in Ashkenazi Jews. The specific mutation is known as R12L.[2, 3] The gene codes for a protein whose exact function is not yet known.

Heredity

Joubert syndrome is inherited in an autosomal recessive manner. A person must inherit a mutation from both parents.

The carrier frequency in those of Ashkenazi Jewish descent appears to be 1:92. There can be variation in the severity of the condition, even within the same family.

Living with the Condition

The combination of issues in this condition can lead to significant disability. Care needs to be taken to deal with the abnormal breathing patterns. It may be necessary to monitor the breathing so apnea can be noted. Supplemental oxygen may be needed. Caffeine may be used to help normalize breathing as well.

Physical therapy can be helpful in dealing with the lack of muscle tone. Hypotonia in the facial area can lead to difficulty swallowing. Speech therapy can help in managing this disordered swallowing. Severe cases of swallowing difficulty may lead to the need for a gastrostomy tube to allow for nutrition without the need to swallow.

Annual assessment of growth, vision, and liver and kidney function are recommended. Those with kidney involvement will need follow-up by a nephrologist. Those with liver involvement will need follow-up with a gastroenterologist.

Sources

M. Parisi and I. Glass, Joubert Syndrome. GeneReviews. http://www.ncbi.nlm.nih.gov/books/NBK1325/

Further Reading

National Institute for Neurological Disorders and Stroke. Joubert Syndrome Information Page. www.ninds.nih.gov/disorders/joubert/joubert. htm

Support Organizations
Joubert Syndrome and Related Disorders Foundation
414 Hungerford Drive, Suite 252
Rockville, MD 20850
Phone: (614) 864-1362
Internet: www.joubertfoundation.com
Joubert Syndrome in the UK
Phone: 01977 709969
Email: info@jsuk.org
Internet: www.jsuk.org

---

1. Dor Yesharim is an organization that provides anonymous testing for Jewish genetic diseases. See the chapter "The Ethics of Genetic Testing" for more details.
2. S. Edvardson, A. Shaag, S. Zenvirt, et al., Joubert Syndrome 2 (JBTS2) in Ashkenazi Jews is associated with a TMEM216 mutation. *Am J Hum Gen* 2010; 86, 93–97.
3. It is a transversion mutation of G>T in codon 3. The gene leads to the production of a protein called *transmembrane protein 216*, where arginine is replaced by leucine. Therefore this mutation is known as R12L.

Limb-Girdle Muscular Dystrophy

Summary

Limb-Girdle Muscular Dystrophy (LGMD) describes a group of diseases of muscle wasting and weakness. These diseases can be caused by a number of different genetic defects. One particular defect, known as *dysferlinopathy*, is more common in Jews whose families originated in Libya. This defect can cause two different clinical syndromes. One, known as *LGMD2B*, first appears in late adolescence with inability to walk on tiptoe and difficulty running and walking. The weakness progresses slowly. The other, known as *Miyoshi myopathy*, presents in young adulthood with muscle weakness mostly in the calf area of the leg. Over a period of years, the weakness and atrophy spread to the thighs and buttocks. The forearms may become mildly weak with a decrease in the strength of the grip, but the rest of the hand muscles continue to be normal. Most individuals with this condition continue to walk until at least their mid-30s. Respiratory and cardiac muscles are generally not involved in either condition.

Historical Background

A relatively high rate of muscular dystrophy in Libyan Jews was first noted in 1991. LGMD2B was first defined as an entity in 1994 and found to be related to a site on chromosome 2. A year later Miyoshi myopathy was linked to the same location. In 1998 the specific gene was identified and found to be mutated in families with both conditions.

Diagnosis of Condition

The condition is suspected with the development of the symptoms of muscle weakness described above. Performance of a blood test for an enzyme known as *creatine phosphokinase* (CPK) will reveal markedly elevated levels that raise the suspicion of some form of muscular dystrophy. Performance of a muscle biopsy can confirm the diagnosis by showing the absence of one of the muscle proteins called *dysferlin*. The specific genetic defect present in Jews whose families originated in Libya can also be tested for.

Genetic Cause

The gene associated with the condition found in Libyan Jews is DYSF, found on the short arm of chromosome 2. A particular mutation, 1624delG, is found in this community.[1]

Heredity

The condition is inherited in an autosomal recessive manner. Both parents need to have the gene for a child to develop the condition. However, since this condition develops in late adolescence or young adulthood, it is possible for someone who unknowingly has it to marry and have children. If he or she marries a carrier, the chances for each pregnancy of having an affected child are 50 percent (not 25 percent, as in autosomal recessive conditions where both parents are unaffected carriers).

The carrier frequency of this gene among Libyan Jews is 1:10. The same mutation is associated with both conditions and both can occur in the same families.

Living with the Condition

Physical therapy is important to help maintain muscle strength and prevent contractures (tightening) of the muscle. Physical therapists can also recommend adaptive equipment such as walkers and crutches to maintain ambulation and proper fitting of wheelchairs when needed.

Extra efforts should be made to prevent obesity, because excess weight affects walking ability.

Sources

E. Gordon, E. Pegoraro, and E. P. Hoffman, Limb-Girdle Muscular Dystrophy Overview. GeneReviews.
http://www.ncbi.nlm.nih.gov/books/NBK1408/
Z. Argov, M. Sadeh, K. Mazor, et al., Muscular dystrophy due to dysferlin deficiency in Libyan Jews: Clinical and genetic features. *Brain*, Vol. 123, No. 6, 1229–37, June 2000.

Suggested Reading

FAQ on LGMD2B/Miyoshi. www.jain-foundation.org/faq.php

Support Organizations
Muscular Dystrophy Association
3300 East Sunrise Drive
Tucson, AZ 85718-3208
Phone: (800) 572-1717
Fax: (602) 529-5300
Email: mda@mdausa.org
Internet: www.mda.org

Muscular Dystrophies Support Group
www.dailystrength.org/c/Muscular-Dystrophies/support-group

---

1. A single G-base deletion at codon 1624 (1624delG), which causes a stop codon to be formed nine base pairs later. The dysferlin produced is thus truncated.

Lipoamide Dehydrogenase Deficiency

Summary
Lipoamide Dehydrogenase (LAD) Deficiency is a condition in which LAD is missing in the mitochondria of the cell.[1, 2] LAD is part of an enzyme complex (pyruvate dehydrogenase) that is needed for energy production. In the presence of this malfunctioning complex, lactic acid builds up in the body, leading to fatigue, especially with exercise. This build-up can also lead to recurrent attacks of vomiting, abdominal pain, and change in mental status accompanied by abnormal liver function. At times these attacks can be fatal. When the condition occurs in the neonatal period, it is generally followed by neurological damage and early demise. When it happens later in childhood, those who have the condition tire easily with exercise but are otherwise well between attacks.

Historical Background
This deficiency of the enzyme as a cause of lactic acidosis (elevated levels of lactic acid) was first reported in 1977 by Dr. B. H. Robinson.[3] Over the following two decades, the association with recurrent attacks of hepatitis was revealed.[4]

Diagnosis of Condition
The condition is suspected in those who present the clinical symptoms described above. It is further suggested by the finding of high blood levels of lactate and pyruvate and the branched chain amino acids leucine, isoleucine, and valine. In mild cases, these elevations will be found only during periods of crisis. The diagnosis is confirmed by demonstrating abnormal enzyme function. This can generally be measured in white blood cells or connective tissue cells; however, in some cases these levels are normal but there are abnormal levels in the muscle cells. Therefore, if the condition is strongly suspected, a muscle biopsy may be done. In a family with a known mutation, or of an ethnic background for which a specific mutation is suspected, such as Ashkenazi Jewish, specific mutations can be tested for.

Genetic Cause
The condition is caused by a defect in a gene found on the long arm of chromosome 7. This gene is called LAD or DLD after the protein for which it codes. Lack of this enzyme in the lymphocytes and muscle cells

leads to build-up of lactic acid and the symptoms of the disease. Two mutations have been found among those of Ashkenazi Jewish descent. The more common one is G229C. Carriage of this mutation was found to be 1:94 among Ashkenazi Jews.

Heredity

The condition is inherited in an autosomal recessive manner. Those with the severe form tend to be homozygous for the same mutation. Those with milder cases tend to have two different mutations.

Living with the Condition

An individually tailored high-fat, low-protein, and low-carbohydrate diet, supplemented with cofactors such as thiamine, biotin, and carnitine, is instituted. When there is a build-up of lactic acid, bicarbonate is given, usually intravenously. Unfortunately, for the neonatal onset of illness, dietary modification generally does not prevent the ongoing significant neurological damage.

Sources

Lipoamide Dehydrogenase Deficiency (E3). Know Your Genes.org. www.knowyourgenes.org/lipoamide-dehydrogenase-deficiency.shtml
R. E. Frye and P. J. Benke. Pyruvate dehydrogenase complex deficiency. eMedicine Pediatrics.
http://emedicine.medscape.com/article/948360-overview
J. Zlotogara, Mendelian Disorders Among Jews.
http://www.health.gov.il/Download/pages/bookjews2011.pdf

Suggested Reading

DLD. Genetics Home Reference.
http://ghr.nlm.nih.gov/gene/DLD

Support Organizations
CLIMB—Children Living with Inherited Metabolic Diseases
Climb Building
176 Nantwich Road
Crewe CW2 6BG
Phone: 0800 652 3181
Fax: 0845 241 2174

Email: fam.svcs@climb.org.uk
Internet: www.climb.org.uk

1. Lipoamide dehydrogenase is a subunit of a number of enzyme complexes, where it is called the E3 subunit. One of these complexes is branched chain alpha-keto acid dehydrogenase (BCKD), which is needed for the breakdown of certain amino acids (see Maple Syrup Urine Disease).
2. The missing enzyme, LAD, that leads to the build-up is also known as *dihydrolipoamide dehydrogenase.*
3. H. B. Robinson, J. Taylor, and W. G. Sherwood, Deficiency of dihydrolipoyl dehydrogenase (a component of the pyruvate and alpha-ketoglutarate dehydrogenase complexes): A cause of congenital chronic lactic acidosis in infancy. *Pediatric Research* 1977:11:1198–1202.
4. N. Barak, D. Huminer, T. Segal, et al., Lipoamide dehydrogenase deficiency: a newly discovered cause of acute hepatitis in adults. *Journal of Hepatology* 1998; 29:482–84.

Maple Syrup Urine Disease

Summary

Maple syrup urine disease (MSUD) is a condition in which the body lacks the enzymes to break down three amino acids (isoleucine, leucine, and valine), collectively known as *branched chain amino acids* (BCAAs) because of their chemical structure. The unchecked build-up of these amino acids, especially leucine, leads to neurological damage. The build-up of isoleucine gives the cerumen (ear wax), urine, and plasma the smell of maple syrup, which is how the condition received its name.

The disease exists in a number of forms. The *classic form* has a rapid onset and, if untreated, can lead to death within the first seven to 10 days of life. People with the classic form generally have less than 3 percent activity of the affected enzyme. In the *intermediate form*, the symptoms will not appear until later in infancy or childhood. In the *intermittent form*, children generally develop normally but will develop vomiting and changes in their mental status when stressed by illness or fasting. The level of enzyme activity among those with the intermediate or intermittent form is generally 3–40 percent of normal.

Historical Background

A family in which four infants died of a neurodegenerative disorder and whose urine had the odor of maple syrup or burnt sugar was described by Dr. John H. Menkes in 1953. In the following years it was discovered that the problem lay with build-up of the branched chain amino acids.

Diagnosis of Condition

The condition is suspected in infants who have the odor of maple syrup in their ear wax in the first day of life, as well as irritability and poor feeding by two to three days of age and worsening symptoms of neurological malfunction within the first week. This or another metabolic condition is suspected when ketones are found in the urine of a newborn.

MSUD can be diagnosed by finding elevated levels of branched chain amino acids in blood plasma. This test can be done between 18 and 24 hours of life. If the answer is equivocal, the test can be repeated between 24 and 36 hours. Because institution of an adapted diet can prevent death and neurological deterioration from this condition, it is now screened for in many locations through the use of dried blood spots generally taken from the infant's heel (along with the standard testing for hypothyroidism and PKU).

Genetic Cause

Proper breakdown of BCAAs involves a cascade of enzymes collectively known as the *branched chain alpha-keto acid dehydrogenase* (BCKAD) complex.[1] BCKAD has four subunits known as E1a, E1b, E2, and E3, each coded by a different gene. A mutation in both alleles of either E1a, E1b, or E2 produces the same clinical picture.[2] A mutation in the fourth component of the BCKAD complex, E3, produces a different clinical picture.[3]

Heredity

MSUD is inherited as an autosomal recessive disease. In order to get the disease one must inherit a mutation from each parent, although not necessarily the same mutation. A number of mutations have been found in each of the three genes that code for each of the subunits.

MSUD is most frequent in the Mennonite population, where the carrier frequency is as high as one in 10. However, at least one mutation has been found to be not infrequent in Ashkenazi Jews. The mutation that is most common in Ashkenazi Jewish patients is R183P in the E1b subunit. A carrier rate of 1:113 for this mutation has been found in this population in the New York area.

Living with the Condition

The key element in the management of this disease is early diagnosis and institution of a special diet that is low in the branched chain amino acids. Blood levels of BCAAs need to be monitored to find the proper balance between allowing enough of these amino acids for proper growth but not enough to overwhelm the system and lead to the neurologic deficit. Careful follow-up is needed by a nutritionist with experience in this condition or a center specializing in metabolic diseases to make sure that the low BCAA diet provides enough essential amino acids and other nutritional needs. Blood levels can be tested on blood dots that are mailed to a regional metabolic center for testing. Monitoring of BCAA levels and adherence to this special diet needs to continue for life.

Special care should be paid to preventing rapid rise of leucine levels at times of stress. A rapid rise of leucine can lead to episodes of brain swelling, potentially leading to coma and death. Parents may be given a home urine test that detects high levels of branched chain alpha-ketoacid (BCKA) and allows starting a "sick day" formula that is even lower in leucine. If the child is unable to tolerate the formula because of vomiting or if there is worsening of his condition, hospitalization is needed for management of the acute crises.

If properly managed, the encephalopathy (brain dysfunction) appears to be reversible. However, young children are likely to have the symptoms of attention deficit disorder and teenagers and adults are likely to suffer from psychological disturbances such as depression or anxiety. Those whose levels are not carefully balanced are likely to develop mental retardation.

Sources
K. A. Strauss, E. G. Puffenberger, and D. H. Morton, Maple Syrup Urine Disease. GeneReviews.
http://www.ncbi.nlm.nih.gov/books/NBK1319/
O. A. Bodamer and B. Lee. Maple Syrup Urine Disease. eMedicine.
http://emedicine.medscape.com/article/946234-overview
J. Zlotogara, Mendelian Disorders Among Jews.
http://www.health.gov.il/Download/pages/bookjews2011.pdf

Suggested Reading
Maple Syrup Urine Disease. Genetics Home Reference.
http://ghr.nlm.nih.gov/condition/maple-syrup-urine-disease

Support Organizations
Maple Syrup Urine Disease Family Support
Phone: (614) 389-2739
Internet: www.msud-support.org
CLIMB—Children Living with Inherited Metabolic Diseases
Climb Building
176 Nantwich Road
Crewe CW2 6BG
Phone: 0800 652 3181
Fax: 0845 241 2174
Email: fam.svcs@climb.org.uk
Internet: www.climb.org.uk

1. This is the second step in the proper breakdown of branched chain amino acids.
2. A mutation on each allele of the first subunit gene, known as BCKDHA, gives rise to a lack of E1a (BCKA decarboxylase alpha subunit) and the disease known as MSUD type 1a. A mutation of each allele of the second subunit gene BCKDHB leads to a lack of E1b (BCKA decarboxylase beta subunit) and MSUD type 1b. A mutation in the gene DBT leads to a lack of the E2 subunit (dihydrolipoyl transacetylase) and MSUD type 2.
3. Carriage of a mutation in the E3 (lipoamide dehydrogenase) component is also found in those of Ashkenazi Jewish descent; see chapter on lipoamide dehydrogenase deficiency.

Megalencephalic Leukoencephalopathy (Vacuolating)

Summary

Megalencephalic leukoencephalopathy (vacuolating) (MLC) is a degenerative neurological condition. It begins with a period of rapid growth of the head circumference starting in the first year of life. The head remains large because of this growth spurt, but the growth rate then becomes normal. This is followed by neurologic difficulties at variable ages. These generally begin with minor motor disability or clumsiness and progress to ataxia (difficulties with balance and gait) and spasticity (stiffness of the muscles). The rate of deterioration is quite variable, but most individuals begin to require a wheelchair during their teenage years. Speech may become difficult and sometimes swallowing becomes problematic. Cognitive functions are affected later and the deficits are relatively mild. Most individuals develop a seizure disorder. Marked changes in the white matter of the brain are seen on MRI (magnetic resonance imaging).

Historical Background

The condition was first reported by Dr. Marjo van der Knaap, a Dutch neurologist, in 1995. Therefore this condition is also known as van der Knaap syndrome.[1]

Diagnosis of Condition

The condition is suspected in children with rapidly progressing head growth. It can be confirmed by the characteristic findings on an MRI of the brain.

Genetic Cause

The condition is linked to the MLC1 gene found on the long arm of chromosome 22. The protein for which this gene codes appears to be part of the cell membrane, but its exact function is not yet known. The condition is relatively common in Jews from Libya living in Israel, where the frequency was tested. One mutation known as c.176G>A[2] has been found in this population. The same mutation is found in a large Jewish family from Turkey, but not among non-Jewish Turks.

Heredity

The form of MLC found in Libyan Jews is inherited in an autosomal recessive manner. Both parents have to be carriers of the mutation. The carrier rate in this community is 1:40.

Living with the Condition

Physical therapy can help improve motor function. Adaptive equipment can assist with mobility. Anti-seizure medications can help control the seizures. Educational assistance can help affected individuals reach their maximal potential.

People with MLC are particularly sensitive to minor head trauma. Therefore it is important that children with this condition wear helmets at most times and avoid activities with a high risk of head trauma. Parental support is needed to help children adjust to having a condition that visibly differentiates them from their peers.

Sources

M. S. Van der Knaap and G. C. Scheper, Megalencephalic Leukoencephalopathy with Subcortical Cysts. GeneReviews.
http://www.ncbi.nlm.nih.gov/books/NBK1535/

Suggested Reading

Megalencephalic leukoencephalopathy with subcortical cysts. Genetics Home Reference.
http://ghr.nlm.nih.gov/condition/megalencephalic-leukoencephalopathy-with-subcortical-cysts

Support Organizations
United Leukodystrophy Foundation (ULF)

2304 Highland Drive
Sycamore, IL 60178
Toll-free: (800) 728-5483
Phone: (815) 895-3211
Fax: (815) 895-2432
Email: office@ulf.org
Internet: www.ulf.org

1. The name *megalencephalic leukoencephalopathy* describes the symptoms. Megalencephaly means "large head," and leukoencephalopathy means "disease of the white matter of the brain."
2. In the gene, G is replaced by A. This leads to p.Gly59Glu.

Metachromatic Leukodystrophy, Late Infantile Type

Summary

Metachromatic Leukodystrophy (MLD) is a *lysosomal storage disease*[1] in which there is a deficiency of the enzyme *arylsulfatase A* (ARSA). This deficiency prevents the breakdown of *sulfatides*, sulfate-containing lipids that are found throughout the body, especially in the nervous system. The build-up of sulfatides in the nervous system damages the lining of the nerves (*myelin*) and leads to a neurological degenerative disease known as a *leukodystrophy*.

Degeneration in MLD is progressive. Deterioration of developmental skills starts between one and two years of age. This is followed by spasms and abnormal posturing and inability to eat orally. In the final stages, which may last for several years, the children are blind, cannot move, do not speak, and do not seem to react to their surroundings. The child generally enters a vegetative state at between three and five years. Death is usually from pneumonia during this stage.

Historical Background

The late infantile form was first described by Dr. Joseph Greenfield in 1933. Therefore, the condition is sometimes called Greenfield's syndrome. In 1959 the term *metachromatic leukodystrophy* was coined, based on a finding on nerve biopsy.[2]

Diagnosis of Condition

The condition is suspected when there is development of neurological difficulties—such as weakness, low muscle tone, clumsiness, frequent falling, or slurred speech—between ages one and two, with progressive degeneration. An MRI will show findings consistent with a leukodystrophy. Reduced levels of ARSA in white blood cells and finding of sulfatides in the urine strengthen the suspicion. However, these findings alone cannot confirm the diagnosis because people can have low levels without the clinical condition. Therefore, molecular genetic testing is needed for definitive diagnosis.

Genetic Cause

The disease is caused by a mutation of the ARSA gene on chromosome 22. The small community of Jews who moved to Israel from Habban,

Yemen, have a high incidence of this condition. All patients from this community have the same mutation.[3]

Heredity

The disease is inherited in an autosomal recessive manner. The carrier frequency in this very closely knit community is 1:6.

Living with the Condition

Untreated, the condition is one of ongoing decline. Physical therapy is important to help prevent contractures (tightening of muscles); lack of contractures makes nursing care easier. Occupational therapy and adaptive equipment can maximize mobility and function as long as possible. Family support is important during a long difficult illness.

Bone marrow transplant prior to the onset of symptoms may prevent the decline. However, the risks associated with the transplant are significant. A laboratory-manufactured form of the enzyme (*metazym*) exists but at the time of this writing is not yet available for purchase.

Sources

A. L. Fluharty, Arylsulfatase A Deficiency. GeneReviews.
http://www.ncbi.nlm.nih.gov/books/NBK1130/
A. K. Ikeda, T. Moore, and R. D. Steiner, Metachromatic leukodystrophy.
eMedicine Pediatrics.
http://emedicine.medscape.com/article/951840-overview
J. Zlotogora, G. Bach, C. Bösenberg, Y. Barak, K. von Figura, and V. Gieselmann. Molecular basis of late infantile metachromatic leukodystrophy in the Habbanite Jews. *Hum Mutat*. 1995; 5:137–43.

Suggested Reading

Metachromatic Leukodystrophy. Genetics Home Reference.
http://ghr.nlm.nih.gov/condition/metachromatic-leukodystrophy

Support Organizations
MLD Foundation

21345 Miles Drive
West Linn, OR 97068
Phone: (800) 617-8387
Fax: (503) 212-0159

Email: info@mldfoundation.org
Internet: http://mldfoundation.org
United Leukodystrophy Foundation (ULF)
2304 Highland Drive
Sycamore, IL 60178
Toll-free: (800) 728-5483
Phone: (800) 728-5483
Fax: (815) 895-2432
Email: office@ulf.org
Internet: www.ulf.org

---

1. Lysosomes are subunits of the cell that contain enzymes that break down substances such as proteins. In lysosomal storage diseases, the lysosomes lack an enzyme needed to break down a particular substance, which then builds up in the lysosome and the cell and causes damage.

2. When the biopsied tissue is subjected to a certain dye, it gives an appearance known as *metachromasia.*

3. The mutation consists of two mutations that generally form the PD (pseudodeficiency) allele that generally leads to low levels of the ARSA enzyme but does *not* lead to disease. However, in this community there is a further mutation in which there is a C to T transition at position 2119, causing a substitution of proline-377 by leucine (P377L). This makes an abnormal enzyme.

Mucolipidosis Type IV

Summary

Mucolipidosis Type IV (shortened at times to ML4 or MLIV) is a neurological disease that results from build-up of lipids and proteins in the *lysosomes* (sacs in the cells whose role is to break down waste products of the cell) due to the lack of the protein *mucolipin-1*. Therefore, this disease is considered one of the *lysosomal storage diseases*.

The severe form of this disease is the most common, especially in those of Ashkenazi Jewish descent. In this form, there is a delay in achievement of motor skills such as sitting, standing, or walking. This delay is generally apparent in the first year of life and most children with the condition do not develop the ability to walk. They are generally intellectually disabled and develop little or no speech. They also tend to have difficulty eating and swallowing. When young, they tend to have low muscle tone, which changes to spasticity (stiffness) as they get older. About 15 percent of patients will undergo neurodegeneration, with loss of motor development already achieved. About 5 percent have an atypical, milder course.

Vision worsens over time. People with the condition tend to develop cataracts (clouding of the lens of the eye) and degeneration of the retina. Most become severely vision impaired or blind by the early teens.

Although this does not cause any symptoms, people with the condition have impaired production of stomach acid. This leads to elevated blood levels of the hormone gastrin, which signals the stomach to produce acid. There tends to be poor absorption of iron from the stomach, leading to anemia.

Length of survival depends on the severity of the condition as well as medical care received. However, most people with this condition live until adulthood, although with a shortened lifespan.

Historical Background

The first case report was published by Dr. E. R. Berman and her colleagues in 1974.[1] An additional three cases were reported the following year.[2]

Diagnosis of Condition

The condition is one of those suspected in infants with severely delayed motor development in the first year. It is further suspected when gastrin levels in the blood are found to be elevated, or typical changes are seen in the lysosomes of cells from skin or conjunctival biopsy. It is confirmed by testing for MCOLN1 mutations.

Genetic Cause

The gene associated with Mucolipidosis IV is known as MCOLN1. This gene, located on chromosome 19, codes for a protein known as *mucolipin-1*. Although the exact purpose of this protein is not yet known, it appears to play a role in the transport of lipids and proteins. The abnormal build-up of the protein and lipids in the cells of the brain and the eye lead to the clinical picture described above.

In persons of Ashkenazi Jewish descent, the disease is usually (95 percent of the time) caused by one of two mutations: c.406-2A>G and g.511_6943del.

Heredity

ML4 disease is inherited in an autosomal recessive manner. To have the disease, one needs to inherit a mutation from both parents. Carriers are not at risk of getting the disorder.

The frequency of carrying any mutation of the MCOLN1 gene in those of Ashkenazi Jewish descent is estimated at between one in 100 and one in 127 people.

Living with the Condition

Physical therapy can help minimize contractures (tightening of muscles) and improve tone and positioning. Orthotics may be helpful as well.

Speech therapy can help provide methods of communication and help assess feeding ability. As feeding becomes more difficult, placement of a gastrostomy tube (feeding tube) can help maintain adequate nutrition and minimize the chances of aspiration.

Eye care is especially important. Lubricants can minimize the pain of corneal erosion, which is especially common in younger children. Strabismus (cross eye) can be treated. Aids for poor vision can help in daily function.

Supplementary iron can be helpful in minimizing the degree of anemia.

Sources
R. Schiffmann, S. A. Slaugenhaupt, J. Smith, and E. Goldin, Mucolipidosis IV. GeneReviews.
http://www.ncbi.nlm.nih.gov/books/NBK1214/

Further Reading
Mucolipidosis Fact Sheet
http://www.ninds.nih.gov/disorders/mucolipidoses/detail_mucolipidoses.htm
Mucolipidosis type IV. Genetics Home Reference.
http://ghr.nlm.nih.gov/condition/mucolipidosis-type-iv/show/print

Support Organizations
Mucolipidosis IV (ML4) Foundation
719 East 17th Street
Brooklyn, NY 11230l
Phone: (718) 434-5067
Fax: (718) 859-7371
Email: ML4www@aol.com
Internet: www.ml4.org
National Mucopolysaccharidoses/Mucolipidoses Society (MPS), Inc.
PO Box 736
Bangor, ME 04402-0736
Phone: (207) 947-1445
Fax: (207) 990-3074
Email: info@mpssociety.org
Internet: www.mpssociety.org
Society for Mucopolysaccharide (MPS) Diseases
MPS House Repton Place White Lion Road
Amersham HP7 9LP
United Kingdom
Phone: 44 0845 389 9901
Email: mps@mpssociety.co.uk
Internet: www.mpssociety.co.uk

National Tay-Sachs and Allied Diseases Association
2001 Beacon Street
Suite 204
Boston, MA 02135
Phone: (800) 90NTSAD (906-8723)
Fax: (617) 277-1034
Email: info@ntsad.org
Internet: www.ntsad.org

1. E. R. Berman, N. Livni, E. Shapira, et al., Congenital corneal clouding with abnormal systemic storage bodies: a new variant of mucolipidosis. *J Pediatr* 1974; 84:519.
2. S. Merin, N. Livni, E. R. Berman, and S. Yatziv, Mucolipidosis IV: Ocular, systemic and ultrastructural findings. *Invest Ophthalmol.* 1975 Jun; 14 (6):437–48.

Nemaline Myopathy

Summary

Nemaline myopathy (NM) is a condition in which there is muscle weakness and low tone, especially in the muscles of the face, neck, upper arms, and thighs. Six different forms of nemaline myopathy have been described but there is significant overlap between them. The symptoms can vary in severity from neonatal respiratory distress and death in the first year (severe congenital NM) to adult onset.

The clinical presentation of the mutation that is more common in Ashkenazi Jews is very low muscle tone (hypotonia), weakness, and feeding difficulties soon after birth or within the first year of life.

Historical Background

The condition was first described in 1963.

Diagnosis of Condition

The condition is suspected when there is local muscle weakness, especially in the face and neck region. Since there are a number of forms of NM, this can present as a newborn with hypotonia, an infant with weakness and feeding difficulties, or an adult with generalized weakness. The suspicion is confirmed if a biopsy of affected muscle contains rod-shaped structures, known as *nemaline bodies*, in the muscle cells that can be seen with an electron microscope. While these rods can be found in other muscle diseases, the combination of the clinical picture and the rods constitutes a definitive diagnosis. Molecular genetic testing can be done in families with a known mutation or in ethnic groups with associated mutations.

Genetic Cause

Defects in six different genes have been associated with nemaline myopathy. They all lead to a disorder in the thin filament proteins of muscle cells. The mutation found in those of Ashkenazi Jewish descent is due to a defect[1] in the NEB gene that codes for the nebulin protein. This gene is found on the long arm of chromosome 2.

Heredity

The form of the disease that has been reported in Ashkenazi Jews is inherited in an autosomal recessive manner. The carrier frequency in this population is approximately 1:100.

Living with the Condition

Low muscle tone in the face and neck can be associated with breathing difficulty and a higher incidence of pneumonia. Therefore, proper treatment for prevention of respiratory infections (such as immunizations to prevent influenza and pneumonia) is important. Special assessment of lung function is needed prior to general anesthesia.

Low tone can also make eating difficult, and those with this condition may need assistance with eating. Placement of a feeding tube may be needed. It is important to monitor growth and nutrition, and high-calorie formulas may be needed. Speech therapy may be of assistance in teaching special feeding techniques and strengthening the facial muscles. It may also be useful with older children if the weakness of the palatal muscles leads to difficulty with speech.

The weakness usually does not progress, or progresses very slowly, and most individuals (especially with the mutation common in Ashkenazi Jews) are able to lead independent, active lives.

Physical therapy can help prevent joint contractures, strengthen muscle, and evaluate whether any adaptive equipment is needed. Prolonged periods of immobility should be avoided since they can exacerbate the muscle weakness.

Sources

K. North and M. M. Ryan, Nemaline Myopathy. GeneReviews.
http://www.ncbi.nlm.nih.gov/books/NBK1288/
J. Zlotogara, Mendelian Disorders Among Jews.
http://www.health.gov.il/Download/pages/bookjews2011.pdf

Suggested Reading

Nemaline Myopathy. Genetics Home Reference.
http://ghr.nlm.nih.gov/condition/nemaline-myopathy
Everybody Is Different. Nemaline Myopathy Support Group Website.
http://www.davidmcd.btinternet.co.uk/Resources/NM_booklet/Everybodys_Different.html. *(This pamphlet is designed especially for children.)*
What Is Nemalin Myopathy? Nemaline Myopathy Support Group Website.
http://www.davidmcd.btinternet.co.uk/Intro/what_is_NM.htm

Support Organizations
Nemaline Myopathy Foundation
PO Box 5937
Round Rock, TX 78683-5937
Phone: (512) 388-7985
A Foundation Building Strength
2450 El Camino Real, Suite 101
Palo Alto, CA 94306
Phone: (650) 320-8000
Email: info@buildingstrength.org
Internet: http://buildingstrength.org
Nemaline Myopathy Support Group
5 Cairnbank Gardens
Penicuik
Midlothian
EH26 9EAUK
Email: davidmcd@hotmail.com
Internet: www.davidmcd.btinternet.co.uk

---

1. The mutation is a 2502 nucleotide deletion that spans exon 55.

Niemann-Pick Disease

Summary

Niemann-Pick disease is a lysosomal storage disease in which the molecules *sphingomyelin* and cholesterol build up in many areas of the body.

There are a number of forms of Niemann-Pick disease. Two types—A and B—have an increased incidence in people of Ashkenazi Jewish descent. Since both forms have been found to be caused by mutations in the same gene, and there are intermediate forms, it is possible that the two types are in fact different ends of a spectrum.

In both forms of the disease, build-up of sphingomyelin and cholesterol in the liver and spleen causes those organs to become markedly enlarged. The effect of the enlarged organs on appetite, as well as swallowing difficulties, can lead to failure to thrive. The enlarged spleen generally removes too many blood cells, which can result in anemia, low levels of white blood cells (which increases the risk of infection), and low levels of platelets (which can lead to bruising and bleeding). In type A there is also accumulation in the brain, leading to neurological degeneration and, generally, death by age 2–3 years. In type B, rapid neurological degeneration does not occur, but the lungs are more likely to be affected. Those with type B generally live through adulthood. Their lifespan will depend on the degree of complications they develop.

Historical Background

In 1914 Dr. Albert Niemann described a girl with an enlarged spleen and swelling who died soon after examination. While the girl had some symptoms of Gaucher disease, Dr. Niemann felt that her condition was a different entity. Starting in 1927, Dr. Ludwig Pick reviewed a number of cases of children with similar symptoms. The biochemical basis of the disease was determined in 1966, and the associated genetic defect was reported in 1997.

Diagnosis of Condition

The condition is suspected when a child is discovered to have an enlarged spleen (in type A this can be as early as three months of age). Those with type A will have problems reaching developmental milestones. As they get older, they lose developmental milestones, become rigid, and do not respond to their surroundings.

Those with type B are generally noticed at first because of an enlarged liver. They may also present with mild findings on chest X-rays done for other reasons.

A particular finding on eye examination will be found in all children with type A and about one-third of children with type B at some point in the course of the disease. It is caused by build-up of the lipids in the ganglion cells of the retina, which makes these cells look very white. This phenomenon is called a *macular halo*. The cells inside the circle are the part of the retina that does not have ganglia and in comparison they can look very red. This is called the *cherry red spot*.

The diagnosis is confirmed by blood testing. White blood cells are tested for the level of the enzyme sphingomyelinase in the white blood cells. A very low level (less than 10 percent of normal) of the enzyme indicates the presence of the disease. Those with type A tend to have lower levels than those with type B. However, it is not possible to predict accurately the severity of the condition by testing for this enzyme. The specific mutation in the gene associated with the illness can then be tested for as well.

Genetic Cause

Those who have Niemann-Pick disease types A and B have a mutation in the SMPD1 gene located on chromosome 11. Therefore, Niemann-Pick disease of these two types is at times called SMPD1-associated. The SMPD1 gene codes for the enzyme *acid sphingomyelinase* (ASM), an enzyme found in the lysosomes, small sacs within the cell whose function is to break down certain products of the cell. Since this enzyme is lacking, the disease is also called *sphingomyelinase* or ASM deficiency. Lack of the enzyme leads to the build-up of sphingomyelin and other lipids, especially cholesterol, in those parts of the body that have many white blood cells, such as the liver, spleen, and bone marrow. In type A it also builds up in the brain. In type B it can also build up in the lungs.

A number of mutations of SMPD1 can cause this condition. In those of Ashkenazi Jewish descent, three mutations account for 90 percent of all cases of type A.[1] Those with type B generally have a 3 base pair deletion (delR608) on both copies of chromosome 11 (homozygous), or have one copy with delR608 and the other with R496L.

Heredity

Niemann-Pick disease is inherited in an autosomal recessive manner; a child must inherit a mutation in the SMPD1 gene (although not necessarily the same one) from each parent in order to be affected. These mutations are found in people of all races, but very rarely. However, the carrier rate of the mutations leading to type A in those of Ashkenazi Jewish ancestry is between 1:80 and 1:100.

The carrier frequency of the mutation leading to type B is lower. Those of Ashkenazi Jewish descent seem also to have a predilection for this mutation, but the incidence and association are less clear.

Living with the Condition

Children with type A generally do not develop past the ability to sit with assistance. They then start to become weaker and less able to do what they once could. Physical and occupational therapy can help maintain muscle function as long as possible and prevent contractures (tightening of muscles). However, ongoing decline is to be expected. Toward the end of their lives, children with this condition become spastic (stiff) and do not relate to their surroundings.

Feeding becomes a major issue over time. The assistance of a dietitian is recommended. Placement of a gastrostomy (feeding) tube may be considered.

Work is under way in the development of potential enzyme replacement therapy,[2] but this is not yet a clinical reality.

Children with type B do not have the neurological deterioration and can live through adulthood. The main concerns for those with type B are:

- *Enlarged spleen*: Children with this condition who have enlarged spleens should avoid participating in contact sports because they are at increased risk of splenic rupture.
- *Low levels of blood components*: Children with this condition will need to have a blood count performed at least annually to follow the status of their blood cells. In severe cases of anemia, splenectomy is considered. However, this is avoided as much as possible since it is likely to worsen the lung disease. Blood transfusions may be needed at times.
- *Growth*: It is important to follow the growth of these children; growth tends to be slower and they tend to be shorter than what would be expected for their family. Eating frequent small meals can help overcome the feeling of fullness that they often have due

to the large liver and spleen. Using high-calorie supplements may help as well.

- *Lungs*: Children with this condition should be evaluated by a lung specialist and followed with lung function tests as recommended.
- *Hyperlipidemia*: Due to the inability to break down cholesterol, persons with this condition are likely to have elevated levels of low-density cholesterol and triglycerides. This places them at increased risk of coronary artery disease. Lipid levels need to be monitored and may require treatment as well.

Women with mild type B have given birth to healthy children, all of whom are by definition carriers of the mutation.

Sources
L. Ierardi-Curto, Niemann-Pick Disease. eMedicine Pediatrics.
http://emedicine.medscape.com/article/951564-overview
R. A. Schwartz, S. A. Centurion, D. Lann, and N. Bartoff, Niemann-Pick Disease. eMedicine Dermatology.
http://emedicine.medscape.com/article/1114349-overview
M. M. McGovern and E. H. Schuchman, Acid Sphingomyelinase Deficiency. GeneReviews.
http://www.ncbi.nlm.nih.gov/books/NBK1370/
E. L. Abel, *Jewish Genetic Disorders*. Jefferson, NC: Macfarland and Co., 2001.

Further Reading
Niemann-Pick Disease. Genetics Home Reference.
http://ghr.nlm.nih.gov/condition/niemann-pick-disease

Support Organizations
National Niemann-Pick Disease Foundation
PO Box 49
Fort Atkinson, WI 53538
Toll-free: (877) CURE-NPC (287-3672)
Phone: (920) 563-0930
Fax: (920) 563-0931
Email: nnpdf@idcnet.com
Internet: www.nnpdf.org

National Tay-Sachs and Allied Diseases Association
2001 Beacon Street
Suite 204
Boston, MA 02135
Email: info@ntsad.org
Internet: www.ntsad.org
Niemann-Pick Disease Group (UK)
11 Greenwood Close
Fatfield, Washington
Tyne and Wear
NE38 8LR
0191 415 6093
Email: Niemann-pick@zetnet.co.uk
Internet: www.niemannpick.org.uk

---

1. L302P: Leucine is replaced by proline at position 302 (or 304 depending on nomenclature used); R496L: Arginine is replaced by leucine at position 496 (or 498 depending on nomenclature) and a single base pair deletion at 330 (or 333) leading to a frame shift.
2. T Kirkegaard, A. G. Roth, N. H. T. Petersen, et al., Hsp70 stabilizes lysosomes and reverts Niemann-Pick disease-associated lysosomal pathology. *Nature* 2010; 463:549-53.

Nonsyndromic Hearing Loss and Deafness

Summary

Deafness from birth occurs in about one in 1,000 births. About half of these cases are inherited, either as part of a syndrome (see, for example, Usher syndrome type I and II) or as an isolated complaint. Those not associated with a syndrome are known as *nonsyndromic congenital deafness*.

This form of hearing loss is moderate to profound. It is present from birth and generally nonprogressive. There are many causes of this condition, but in the Ashkenazi Jewish population, most cases are associated with mutations in one particular gene.

Historical Background

The condition of deafness has been known since antiquity. The Mishna has many discussions about the halachic status of the deaf (see the chapter on Halachic Living with Genetic Conditions). Many different genes have been associated with inherited congenital deafness. An association of the majority of these conditions with mutations in the connexin-producing genes has been known since approximately the year 2000.

Diagnosis of Condition

The condition is suspected when a child fails to develop speech at the appropriate age. With the onset of recommendations for newborn hearing screening,[1] it is likely to be diagnosed soon after birth. In families known to have the condition, testing should be done soon after birth to allow for early intervention.

Genetic Cause

In those of Ashkenazi Jewish descent, this condition has been linked to the GJB2 gene found on the long arm of chromosome 13. This gene codes for the protein connexin 26. This protein forms channels that allow for molecules to pass between cells in the inner ear.

The most common mutation in this population is 167delT, which is rare in other populations.[2] The mutation 30delG,[3] which is the most common in those of northern European ancestry, has also been found, but less frequently.

Heredity

The mutation causing the condition in the Ashkenazi Jewish population is inherited in an autosomal recessive manner. The carrier rate of the c.167delT mutation in the Ashkenazi Jewish population is approximately 1:13.

Living with the Condition

Hearing aids amplify sound and enable a person to take advantage of any hearing he or she does have. For some children, cochlear implants may be appropriate. Early implementation is important for the development of speech..

Speech and language therapy should be given from an early age to promote proper communication skills. Specialists can help recommend adaptations to the school and work environment to maximize independent functioning. Consultation with an educational institution for the deaf is important to develop an individualized approach to the communication skills needed (e.g., lip reading, sign language).

Other devices are available to assist with hearing in specific situations such as classroom video presentations and telephones. Signaling devices are available to convert sounds to visual signals and allow the person to detect things such as an alarm clock or a baby crying.

Any other middle ear diseases, such as ear infections, should be treated to prevent the additive effect of the hearing loss that accompanies these diseases.

Sources

R. J. Morell, J. K. Hung, L. J. Hood, et al., Mutations in the connexin 26 gene (G2B2) among Ashkenazi Jews with nonsyndromic recessive deafness. *N Eng J Med* 1998; 339:1500–1505.
R. J. H. Smith and G. V. Camp, Nonsyndromic hearing loss and deafness, DFNB1. GeneReviews.
http://www.ncbi.nlm.nih.gov/books/NBK1272
S. A. Moody-Antonio and B. Strassnick, Inner Ear, Genetic Sensorineural Hearing Loss. eMedicine Otolaryngology and Facial Plastic Surgery.
http://emedicine.medscape.com/article/856116-overview

Suggested Reading

Nonsyndromic Deafness. Genetics Home Reference.
http://ghr.nlm.nih.gov/condition/nonsyndromic-deafness.

Support Organizations
Alexander Graham Bell Association for the Deaf and Hard of Hearing
3417 Volta Place, NW
Washington, DC 20007
Phone: (202) 337-5220
TTY: (202) 337-5221
Fax: (202) 337-8314
Email: info@agbell.org
Internet: http://nc.agbell.org/netcommunity/page.aspx?pid=348
Hearing Loss Association of America
7910 Woodmont Avenue, Suite 1200
Bethesda, MD 20814
Phone: (301) 657-2248
Internet: www.hearingloss.org

www.deafdoc.org is a site written by a family physician who is herself
hearing impaired.

Our Way for the Deaf and Hard of Hearing
The National Jewish Council for Disabilities
11 Broadway, 13th Floor
New York, NY 10004
Phone: (212) 613-8229
Fax: (212) 613-0796
Email: njcd@ou.org

---

1. Joint Committee on Infant Hearing. Joint Committee on Infant Hearing Year
2000, Position Statement: Principles and Guidelines for Early Hearing Detection
and Intervention Programs. *Pediatrics* 2000; 106:798–817.
2. This means that thymine is deleted from codon 167. This leads to a defective
connexin protein.
3. This means that guanine is missing from codon 30. This too leads to a defective
connexin protein.

Tay-Sachs Disease

Summary

Tay-Sachs is one of a group of genetic diseases called *lysosomal storage diseases*. It results from lack of the enzyme B-hexosaminidase A (HEX-A), which is found in the lysosomes (small sacs within cells, whose function is to break down certain products of the cell). When this enzyme is not functional, molecules called GM_2 *gangliosides* build up in the cells of the nervous system including in the brain, and this build-up eventually causes the symptoms of Tay-Sachs.

In the most common, classic, form of Tay-Sachs, the infant will initially show normal patterns of development. Generally between three and six months of life there are signs of decreasing development. The infant will eventually develop blindness, macrocephaly (an enlarged head), hypotonia (low muscle tone, floppiness), spasticity (stiffness), hyperreflexia (overly brisk reflexes), an increased startle response, and eventually seizures.[1, 2] In most cases death from pneumonia will occur by two to eight years of age.[3, 4, 5] Other forms of the disease are discussed in the Genetic Cause section.

Historical Background

The condition was first described by two different physicians. In 1881 Dr. Warren Tay, an ophthalmologist, described the eye findings of a "cherry red spot."[6] Dr. Bernard Sachs, a neurologist, indicated the hereditary nature of the condition in 1896.

Diagnosis of Condition

The condition is suspected in infants who are normal at birth and begin to show signs of developmental regression at three to six months of age. It can be confirmed by measurement of low levels of beta-hexosaminidase A enzyme levels in the serum or white blood cells, together with the presence of normal or elevated beta-hexosaminidase B (a similar enzyme). The specific mutation can be determined for purposes of genetic counseling.

Genetic Cause

The most frequent DNA mutation leading to Tay-Sachs disease in Ashkenazi Jews (80 percent) is a four-base pair insertion in exon 11 of the HEXA gene found on the long arm of chromosome 15. This mutation is found in 8 to 32 percent of non-Jewish carriers. This insertion leads to formation of an unstable mRNA, which falls apart and is not able to make a functioning hexosaminidase enzyme. When the enzyme is completely missing, the child will be affected with the classic form of Tay-Sachs and is expected to die in early childhood. A different mutation at the same location will cause partial deficiency of the enzyme, later onset of the condition, and life prolonged to the mid-teens. Mutation in another location[7] accounts for 13 to 33 percent of cases of classic Tay-Sachs in Ashkenazi Jewish families and is almost never found in non-Jewish carriers.

There is an additional mutation[8] that occurs in Ashkenazi Jews, which leads to low enzyme levels that are detected in enzymatic testing but does not lead to clinical disease. When the third mutation is paired with one of the first two, the person can develop late-onset Tay-Sachs, a gradual deterioration of neurological function, half of the time coupled with psychiatric manifestations such as depression or psychosis, with survival to ages 60 to 80.

Heredity

Tay-Sachs disease is an autosomal recessive disease. Carriers of the disease are not at risk of getting the disorder. A mutation needs to be inherited from both parents.

The frequency of carrying any mutation of the gene in those of Ashkenazi Jewish descent is estimated at between one in 25 and one in 30 people. The frequency of the disease used to be one in 3,600 Ashkenazi Jewish births, but because of carrier testing, the rate has been reduced by more than 90 percent.[9] No cases have been reported in the ultra-Orthodox community in Israel since the onset of Dor Yesharim screening.[10]

Jews of North African origin carry a number of mutations in this gene at a rate of approximately 1:100. Jews of other non-Ashkenazi origin carry mutations at rates similar to the non-Jewish population—approximately 1:300.

Living with the Condition

Treatment of the infantile form is primarily supportive until expected demise. Attention needs to be given to nutrition and hydration and the control of seizures.

Those with the late onset form primarily need assistance in proper diagnosis, since this lesser known condition may be confused with other neurological or psychiatric conditions. It is important to realize that the neurological or psychiatric symptoms are a manifestation of late onset Tay-Sachs, since specific medications may be more appropriate for use in these cases.[11]

Sources
M. M. Kaback, Hexosaminidase A Deficiency. GeneReviews.
http://www.ncbi.nlm.nih.gov/books/NBK1218/

Further Reading
Tay-Sachs Information Page, National Institute of Neurological Disorders and Stroke.
http://www.ninds.nih.gov/disorders/taysachs/taysachs.htm
Tay-Sachs Disease. Genetics Home Reference.
http://ghr.nlm.nih.gov/condition/tay-sachs-disease
Learning about Tay-Sachs, National Human Genome Research Institute.
www.genome.gov/page.cfm?pageID=10001220

Support Organizations
National Tay-Sachs and Allied Diseases Association
2001 Beacon Street
Suite 204
Boston, MA 02135
Phone: (800) 90NTSAD (906-8723)
Fax: (617) 277-1034
Email: info@ntsad.org
Internet: www.ntsad.org

---

1. J. A. F. Filho and B. E. Shapiro, Tay-Sachs Disease. *Arch Neurology*; Vol. 61, September 2004, pp. 1466 –68.
2. V. Reid Sutton, MD, Tay-Sachs disease screening and counseling families at risk for metabolic disease, *Obstet Gynecol Clin N Am* 2002; 29:287–96.
3. J. Charrow, Ashkenazi Jewish Genetic Disorders. *Familial Cancer*. 2004; 3 (3–4):201–6.
4. L. Jorde, J. Carey, M. Bamshad, and R. White. *Medical Genetics* 3rd ed., St. Louis, MO: Mosby, 2006–2007.
5. B. Bembi et al., Substrate reduction therapy in the infantile form of Tay-Sachs disease. *Neurology*, 2006; 66; 278–80.
6. This is caused by build-up of the lipids in the ganglion cells of the retina, which makes these cells look very white; this effect is called a macular halo. The cells

inside the circle are the part of the retina that does not have ganglia and in comparison it can look very red and is called the "cherry red spot."

7. Transversion of G to C in intron 12.

8. G to A transition in exon 7 that changes amino acid 269 from glycine to leucine.

9. M. M. Kabbak. Population-based genetics screening for reproductive counseling: the Tay-Sachs experience. *Eur J Peds* 2000; 159:S192–5.

10. E. Broide, M. Zeigler, J. Eckstein, and G. Bach, Screening for carriers of Tay-Sachs Disease in the ultraorthodox Ashkenazi Jewish community in Israel. *Am J Med Gen* 1993; 47:213–15.

11. O. Neudorfer, E. H. Kolodny Late-onset Tay-Sachs Disease. *IMAJ* 2004; 6:107–11.

Thalassemias

Melissa Meyers[1]

Thalassemia is a condition in which individuals are missing part of the hemoglobin molecule, the component of the red blood cell that binds to oxygen. Each hemoglobin molecule is made up of an iron carrying molecule (*heme*) and four amino acid chains that make a protein known as *globulin*. In adults, the four chains consist of a pair of *alpha chains* and a pair of *beta chains*.[2] Thalassemias are diseases in which some or all of these chains are missing. As a result, the defective hemoglobin is less able to carry the oxygen to all parts of the body, leading to lack of energy. The body attempts to produce more hemoglobin to make up for what is missing, leading to enlarged organs such as the liver and spleen.

Thalassemia is named from the Greek word *thalassa*, meaning "the sea," because the disease was first noted among people living near the Mediterranean Sea. In later years the constellation of thalassemias has been noted in other areas such as Asia and Africa.

The thalassemias are one of a number of genetic diseases affecting the red blood cell. Such diseases are more common in people from historically malaria-endemic areas, where carrying a mutation confers a protective effect from the mosquito-borne disease. These areas include the Middle East.

Alpha Thalassemia
Summary

Alpha thalassemia is the condition in which between one and four of the alpha genes needed to produce the two alpha chains are missing. This absence results in the production of hemoglobin with more beta chains than alpha chains. If the hemoglobin molecule produced has four beta globulin chains, it is called *hemoglobin H*. This form of hemoglobin is unstable and tends to precipitate (come out of solution from the liquid portion of the cell) in the red blood cell and damage its membrane. The amount of precipitation rises with the age of the red blood cell and thus these cells tend to have a lifespan that is shorter than the normal 120 days.

Those who are missing only one gene are called *silent carriers* and are generally asymptomatic. The condition of those with two missing genes is called *alpha thalassemia trait*. They generally are asymptomatic or have mild anemia. Those with three missing genes produce measurable levels of hemoglobin H and are likely to have more significant anemia and enlarged organs. They may also develop frequent infections, have poor healing of wounds, and have a greater risk of blood clots. In severe cases, they may develop heart failure by age 30. This condition is known as *hemoglobin H disease*. The most severe form of the disease is known as *Bart's syndrome.* This occurs when the body cannot produce any alpha globin chains. Bart's syndrome leads to severe anemia in utero, which generally results in heart failure and fetal death.

Diagnosis of Condition

Alpha thalassemia is suspected in cases of anemia with small red blood cells (microcytic anemia) among patients from parts of the world where this condition is common. In older children and adults it can be confirmed by finding collections of precipitated hemoglobin H (inclusion bodies) on microscopic examination of stained red blood cells. A blood test known as *hemoglobin electrophoresis* can show the presence of he-moglobin H, also known as *Bart's hemoglobin*. Carriers generally have about 1–2 percent of this abnormal hemoglobin, a level that is at times too low to be seen on this test. Those with a level of more than four percent are considered to be affected by the condition. Those with hemoglobin H disease will have 20–40 percent. This test can be done on umbilical cord blood. Testing DNA for specific mutations is possible in those with a sug-gestive family history.

Genetic Cause

Two linked genes coding for alpha globin (HBA1 and HBA2) are found on the short arm of chromosome 16. A child receives two pairs of these genes (a total of four genes), two from each parent. A defect in any one of these four genes can lead to the disease. Among Jews, the most common cause is a 3,700-base deletion. Yemenite Jews have been found to have a unique deletion of 39,000 bases that include two genes.

Heredity

In order to have symptomatic alpha thalassemia, a person needs to have at least two mutations. These can be either multiple mutations on one copy of chromosome 16 (inherited from one parent) or one mutation on each of the two copies of the chromosome (each inherited from a differ-ent parent). It is therefore possible for this to be inherited as an autosomal dominant condition, with the child receiving two mutations from the same parent.[3] These cases tend to be milder. If each parent has a mutation in only one gene, the disease is inherited as an autosomal recessive condition.

The carrier rate in Yemenites is estimated at four percent and is somewhat lower among Iraqi Jews. About 1:80 Kurdish Jews are affected by the condition (primarily as silent carriers). Isolated mutations have been found in Ashkenazi Jews as well, with an estimated frequency of 5 percent.

Living with the Condition

Those with mild anemia generally need no treatment. Knowing that one is a carrier of alpha thalassemia can help explain the low level of hemoglobin and prevent unnecessary treatment with iron. Knowing that one has the mutation is important only for purposes of avoiding conceiving children who might be more severely affected.

Those with hemoglobin H diseases need appropriate management of the complications listed above. Blood transfusions are generally needed to treat the anemia. Frequent blood transfusions can lead to iron overload and the need for *chelation therapy*, giving medications that can bind the excess iron and allow for its excretion. Removal of a markedly enlarged spleen is often necessary by the second or third decade of life. Some severe cases may lead to heart failure and early death.

If a fetus is diagnosed with Bart's syndrome, the mother is at high risk of developing high blood pressure and a dangerous condition known as *preeclampsia*.[4] Fetal death in utero (after 33 weeks gestation) or within a few hours of birth is generally expected. The few children who have survived past birth had significant anatomical and developmental abnormalities. Recent developments in neonatal and newborn care have not greatly affected the survival of these infants.

Sources

S. A. Bleibel, R. J. Leonard, J. L. Jones-Crawford, et al., Alpha Thalassemia, eMedicine Hematology.
http://emedicine.medscape.com/article/206397-overview
R. Galanello and A. Cao, Alpha-Thalassemia, GeneReviews.
http://www.ncbi.nlm.nih.gov/books/NBK1435/
L. Shalmon, C. Kirschmann, and R. Zaizov, Alpha-thalassemia Genes in Israel: Deletion and Nondeletional Mutations in Patients of Various Origins. *Hum Hered* 1996; 46 (1):9–15.
E. P. Vichinsky, Alpha Thalassemia Major – New Mutations, Intrauterine Management, and Outcomes. *Hematology* 2009; 35–41.

Further Reading
Sephardic Jewish Genetic Diseases Resource.
http://www.victorcenters.org/sephardi-info.cfm
Alpha Thalassemia. Genetics Home Reference.
http://ghr.nlm.nih.gov/condition/alpha-thalassemia

Beta Thalassemia
Summary
     Beta thalassemia occurs when there is difficulty in the production of
beta chains. The difficulty can be an inability to produce beta chains[5] or
production of a decreased amount of beta chains.[6] If there is an inability
to produce enough beta chains, the hemoglobin molecule will use other
chains as well. When alpha chains are substituted for beta chains, then
the hemoglobin is unstable and can precipitate and damage the cell membrane. These defective red blood cells are broken down by the spleen,
leading to anemia and an enlarged spleen. In the face of reduced or absent
beta chains, the body will sometimes use a different chain known as a
delta chain. Hemoglobin that is made up of alpha chains and delta chains
is known as *Hemoglobin A2.*
     This condition exists in three clinical forms: major, intermedia, and
minor. *Beta thalassemia major* usually presents between the ages of two
months and two years with a variety of symptoms including jaundice and
yellowed eyes; enlarged heart, spleen, and liver; misshapen and fragile
bones; and poor growth and weight gain known as "failure to thrive."
Affected children develop a severe form of anemia, which may be life-
threatening. The build-up of iron in the body due to increased absorption
as the body attempts to fight the anemia can damage the heart and the
endocrine system. Death at a young age results from this condition unless
the child is treated with transfusions and chelation therapy or a blood-
producing cell transplantation. In the past, this transplantation was of the
bone marrow. Currently, it can be done with cells from umbilical cord
blood instead.
     Patients suffering from *beta thalassemia intermedia* experience milder
symptoms that may present in later childhood or adolescence. Symptoms
include a milder form of anemia, growth retardation, and bone weakness.
These children often do not need transfusions. However, they still may
need chelation therapy to prevent iron overload, since their bodies absorb
more iron than normal from the food they eat to try to compensate for their
anemia.

Individuals who have only one abnormal gene often have *beta thalassemia minor*, a microcytic anemia that generally does not need treatment. It is important to recognize thalassemia minor so it is not confused with iron deficiency anemia and treated unnecessarily with iron, and so the person realizes that he is a carrier for the purpose of avoiding conceiving children who are more seriously affected.

Historical Background

Dr. Thomas Cooley, an American pediatrician in the early 1920s, described this condition among immigrants from Italy. For this reason it is also at times called Cooley's anemia.

Diagnosis of Condition

Diagnostic screening of newborns is standard in those areas of the world with a high incidence of the condition, such as the Mediterranean, North Africa, the Middle East, and Asia. When not diagnosed in the newborn period, beta thalassemia major is suspected in cases of anemia with an enlarged liver and spleen, or jaundice or heart failure. The trait is suspected in patients with mild microcytic anemia, a condition in which the red blood cells are smaller than normal. Confirmation is done by testing for elevated levels of hemoglobin A2 (Hb A2).

Genetic Cause

Beta thalassemia is caused by one or more of many possible mutations in the HBB gene on the short arm of chromosome 11, which codes for the beta globin components of hemoglobin.

Heredity

Beta thalassemia is most commonly inherited in an autosomal recessive pattern, where both parents carry the mutation.[7] A child of two carriers has a 1:4 chance of having beta thalassemia major. There is a 1:2 chance of having thalassemia minor.

Carrier frequency among Iraqi and Iranian populations has been reported as 1:6.

Living with the Condition

Anemia causes fatigue as the lack of a normal beta globin chain impairs the ability of the red blood cells to adequately transport oxygen to the body. Ongoing attempts of the body to make more hemoglobin in the liver and the spleen and bones of the skull, in addition to the bone marrow of the arms and legs, lead to enlargement of those organs. The main goal of treatment is to compensate for the defective hemoglobin by supplementing with healthy blood cells through frequent transfusions. This treatment, which involves frequent insertions of intravenous catheters, provides normal cells capable of transporting oxygen effectively. It generally also suppresses the body's need to compensate for the anemia as well as reduce enlargement of the liver and spleen. However, a side effect of transfusions (in addition to risks of blood-borne diseases) is the build-up of large amounts of iron, which is part of the hemoglobin molecule. Chelation therapy, an iron-removing process, is needed to prevent the dangerous accumulation of the metal. Removal of the enlarged spleen may be needed. However, removal of this organ, especially in younger children, makes the individual susceptible to a number of infections.

If a matched donor can be found, transplantation can cure the disease by providing a source of production of normal red blood cells. However, the transplantation procedure and the ongoing suppression of the immune system can have a number of serious side effects.

Sources
K. Takeshita, Thalassemia, Beta. eMedicine Hematology.
http://emedicine.medscape.com/article/206490
A. Cao and R. Galanello, Beta-Thalassemia. GeneReviews.
http://www.ncbi.nlm.nih.gov/books/NBK1426/

Further Reading
Sephardic Jewish Genetic Diseases Resource.
http://www.victorcenters.org/sephardi-info.cfm
Cooley's Anemia Foundation. http://www.cooleysanemia.org/updates/
pdf/Beta_Thalassemia.pdf

Support Organizations
Cooley's Anemia Foundation
330 Seventh Avenue, #900
New York, NY 10001
Phone: (800) 522-7222
Email: Info@cooleysanemia.org
Internet: www.cooleysanemia.org

1. Melissa Meyers is a student at the Sackler School of Medicine in Tel Aviv, and is currently in the clinical portion of her training. In addition to medicine, Meyers has an interest in bioethics and halacha. She has also studied at Pardes and the Schlesinger Institute.

2. Infants have other chains that make fetal hemoglobin.

3. Because of the variability of expression of this condition, the parent may or may not know that he or she has alpha thalassemia.

4. A combination of high blood pressure and protein in the urine. Severe cases can lead to eclampsia, a life-threatening condition that includes seizures. The risk to a mother's life may lead to consideration of abortion. In a case such as this where there is significant risk to the mother and minimal chance of survival of the fetus, abortion is permissible and may very well be mandated. As circumstances vary, an individual halachic ruling should be sought.

5. This is known as B^0.

6. This is known as B^+.

7. A dominant form has been reported but it is quite rare.

Usher Syndromes

Introduction

Usher syndrome is a combination of deafness and a form of progressive visual difficulty known as *retinitis pigmentosa*. Since 1989, Usher syndrome has been divided into three types (I, II, and III), differentiated by the time of onset of the deafness.

Historical Background

In 1914 a Scottish ophthalmologist, Dr. Charles Usher, conducted a study of deafness in people with visual problems in Britain and reported his data analysis of 69 cases. For this reason, the syndrome bears his name. It is interesting to note that in 1861 a number of cases of combined retinitis pigmentosa and hearing difficulty had been reported by a German ophthalmologist, Dr. Albrecht von Graefe, in the Jewish population of Berlin. For this reason, the condition is sometimes called Graefe-Usher syndrome. A high frequency was also reported in the Jewish community of Vienna in 1907.

Usher Syndrome Type I
Summary

In Usher syndrome type I, the deafness is congenital, present at birth or at least before the child has learned to speak. The visual difficulty begins later, generally in the early teenage years. Type I is also accompanied by problems in the function of the inner ear (vestibula), which is responsible for balance.

Diagnosis of Condition

The condition is suspected when there is congenital deafness. Children with type I also tend to walk late (18–24 months) because of their balance difficulties. Because the visual deterioration develops later in life, the syndrome may not actually be suspected until there is the combination of deafness and retinitis pigmentosa. However, at least in populations where the genetic mutation is known, such as those of Ashkenazi Jewish descent, it can be predicted earlier through targeted molecular genetic analysis looking for the suspected mutation(s).

Genetic Cause

A number of genes are associated with Usher type I. It has been sub-divided according to the genetic mutation. The subtype associated with those of Ashkenazi Jewish descent is 1F. The gene associated with this subtype is called PCDH15 and is located on the long arm of chromosome 10. It codes for a protein called protocadherin-15.[1] This protein is involved in the development of various parts of the brain as well as the hair-like cells of the ear known as the *cilia*. The mutation that occurs in those of Ashkenazi Jewish descent is R245X.[2]

The subtype of Usher type I that occurs among Jews from North Africa is type 1B. This is caused by a mutation in the MYO7A gene found on the long arm of chromosome 11. This gene codes for a protein known as myosin VIIA, which appears to play a role in the development of hair cells in the cochlea of the ear. The mutation in this gene, known as Ala826Thr,[3] is frequently found among Jewish patients from both Algeria and Morocco. In addition, among patients of Moroccan Jewish origin, two other mutations were also present: Gly214Arg and 2065delC.

Heredity

Usher syndrome of both type 1B and type 1F is inherited in an autosomal recessive pattern. To get either condition, one needs to inherit a mutation for that subtype from each parent. Since type 1B and type 1F are on different genes, inheriting one mutation on each of these two separate genes would most likely not cause the condition.[4]

The carrier rate of the mutation in those of Ashkenazi Jewish descent is estimated to be approximately between 1:20 and 1:40. The carrier frequency of the various mutations among Jews from North Africa has not yet been reported.

Usher Syndrome Type II
Summary

In Usher syndrome type II, the moderate to severe deafness begins early in life but after speech has been acquired. Hearing loss is generally moderate in the low frequencies but severe to profound in the higher frequencies. The loss does not get worse as the person ages. The visual difficulty begins later, generally in the early teenage years. There are no problems in the function of the inner ear (vestibula), which is responsible for balance, in type II.

Diagnosis of Condition

The disease is suspected when there is onset of deafness in infancy that is followed by visual difficulties typical of retinitis pigmentosa, such as night blindness and tunnel vision. The condition can be confirmed by molecular genetic testing.

Genetic Cause

Most cases of Usher syndrome type II are associated with defects in the USHA2A gene found on the long arm of chromosome 1. This gene codes for *usherin*, which is part of a complex of proteins that also includes the products of other genes associated with Usher syndrome. Lack of any one of these proteins leads to degeneration of the cochlea and retina.

A number of mutations to the USHA2A gene have been reported in families of non-Ashkenazi Jewish descent. The following four account for 64 percent of all mutations in this population:

1. In families originating from North Africa (Morocco and Tunisia), c.1000C>T. The carrier frequency for this mutation was slightly less than 1:100 in this population.
2. In families originating from Buchara, c.12067-2A>G. The carrier rate has not been determined.
3. In families from Iraq and Iran, a frame shift mutation, c.239-240insGTAC. The carrier frequency is not yet known.
4. In families from Iraq, c.2209C>T mutation. The carrier frequency is not yet known.

Heredity

The condition is inherited in an autosomal recessive manner. Inheriting a mutation from each parent, even if not the same mutation, can lead to this condition.

Usher Syndrome Type III

Summary

In Usher syndrome type III, the timing of the onset of hearing loss and visual defects is variable. The hearing loss begins in early childhood, generally after the development of speech, and is progressive. There is also visual loss. Sometimes the visual loss precedes the hearing loss.

Diagnosis of Condition

The condition is suspected when there are signs of hearing loss (e.g., speaking abnormally loudly, turning up the volume of the television). The visual loss begins with difficulty with night vision. Testing for the genetic mutation can help differentiate the types of Usher syndrome, especially in the Ashkenazi Jewish population, where the condition is associated with specific genetic mutations.

Genetic Cause

The gene associated with Usher syndrome type III is USH3 on the long arm of chromosome 3. A number of mutations of this gene have been reported. The one that has been detected in those of Ashkenazi Jewish descent is known as N48K.[7] This mutation disrupts the translation of the protein clarin I, which is found in the cochlea and retina and whose exact function is unknown.[8]

Heredity

Usher syndrome type III is inherited in an autosomal recessive pattern. The carrier frequency of this mutation is approximately 1:221 in the Ashkenazi Jewish population.

Living with the Condition

For all those with Usher syndrome, help should be given for the hearing difficulties. Hearing aids may be of assistance for those with moderate hearing loss. Intervention for profound hearing loss may include cochlear implants.

Assistive devices for visual difficulty will be needed as well. Receiving educational interventions devised for the deaf-blind is important. Computer Sciences for the Blind (CSB) has a computer program that can translate written Hebrew texts into voice and Braille. They can be contacted at (718) 837-4549 or www.computersciences.org.

It is important that individuals with this condition be followed by an ophthalmologist to ensure that their vision is not further compromised by treatable conditions such as cataracts.

For those with Usher syndrome type I, involvement in sports can help preserve coordination and balance. Swimming needs to be carefully supervised, since one of the deficiencies of vestibular function is losing the sense of "which way is up."

In those of Ashkenazi Jewish descent, Usher syndrome of all types is common enough that all children with hearing loss should be followed by an ophthalmologist and those with signs of retinitis pigmentosa should have their hearing checked.

Sources
J. B. Keats and J. Lentz, Usher Syndrome Type I, GeneReviews.
http://www.ncbi.nlm.nih.gov/books/NBK1265/
J. B. Keats and J. Lentz, Usher Syndrome Type II, GeneReviews.
http://www.ncbi.nlm.nih.gov/books/NBK1341/
S. L. Ness, T. Ben Yosef, A. Bar-Lev, et al., Genetic homogeneity and phenotypic variability among Ashkenazi Jews with Usher syndrome type III. *J Med Genet* 2003; 40:767–72.

Suggested Reading
Usher Syndrome. Genetics Home Reference.
http://ghr.nlm.nih.gov/condition/usher-syndrome
Usher Syndrome: New insights lead to Earlier Treatment. NIDCD Health Information. http://www.nidcd.nih.gov/health/hearing/usher.asp

Support Organizations
Usher Syndrome Foundation
10601 Twilight Drive
St. Louis, MO 63128
Phone: (314) 283-1227
Internet: www.ushersyndromefoundation.org
Usher Family Support
11435 Cranhill Drive
Owing Mills, MD 21117
Phone: (800) 683-5555
Helen Keller National Center for Blind-Deaf Youths and Adults
141 Middle Neck Road
Sands Point, NY 11050
Phone: (516) 994-8900, Ext. 254
Email: hkncinfo@hknc.org
Internet: www.hknc.org

National Consortium on Deaf Blindness
Phone: (800) 438-9376
Fax: (503) 838-8150
Email: info@nationaldb.org
Internet: www.nationaldb.org
JBI International (formerly **Jewish Braille Institute**)
110 East 30th Street
New York, NY 10016
Phone: (800) 433-1531
Fax: (212) 689-3692
Internet: www.jbilibrary.org
Our Way for the Deaf and Hard of Hearing
The National Jewish Council for Disabilities
11 Broadway, 13th Floor
New York, NY 10004
Phone: (212) 613-8229
Fax: (212) 613-0796
Email: njcd@ou.org
Internet: www.njcd.org

---

1. T. Ben Yosef, S. L. Ness, A. C. Madeo, et al., A mutation of PCDH15 among Ashkenazi Jews with the Type 1 Usher Syndrome. *N Eng J Med* 2003; 348:1664–90.
2. Replacement of arginine at position 245 leads to a stop codon and a shortened, nonfunctional protein.
3. Threonine replaces alanine at position 826.
4. Although this situation has not yet, to the best of our knowledge, been reported in the medical literature.
5. At position 1000 cytosine is replaced by thiamine. This change results in arginine being replaced by tryptophan. Therefore, this mutation is also known as p.R334W.
6. This mutation is also called p.T80fsX28.
7. A substitution of lysine for asparagine.
8. S. L. Ness, T. Ben Yosef, A. C. Madeo, et al., Genetic homogeneity and phenotypic variability among Ashkenazi Jews with Usher syndrome type III. *J Med Genet* 2003; 40:767–72.

Other Genetic Diseases

Down Syndrome

Summary

Down syndrome is the most common chromosomal disorder, as well as the most common cause of mental retardation. It is a condition of specific physical findings and mild to moderate mental retardation. Individuals with Down syndrome tend to look more like each other than they look like their siblings. The facial features include slanted eyes, a small nose with a flat nasal bridge, and an open mouth with a tendency for the relatively large tongue to protrude. They have characteristic folds on the palms of their hands, known as *simian creases*. About half of the children with this condition are born with congenital heart lesions.

Historical Background

In 1866 the syndrome was described by Dr. John Langdon Haydon Down, an English physician, and thus the common terminology for the condition bears his name. The link of the condition to three copies of chromosome 21 was discovered in 1959.

Diagnosis of Condition

The condition is suspected when an infant is born with the typical physical findings of the syndrome. It is confirmed by performance of a *karyotype*—testing the number of chromosomes found in a cell, generally done on white blood cells.

Very often, the condition has already been suspected during prenatal care.[1]

Genetic Cause

Nondisjunction (failure of a chromosome pair to separate) of chromosome 21 in the egg or sperm results in one extra copy of the chromosome being inherited. Therefore, Down syndrome is also known as *trisomy 21*. When the extra pair appears in only some of a person's cells, this condition is known as *mosaicism*. Those with mosaicism may be less affected by the syndrome.

238

Heredity

Almost all cases are spontaneous events related to nondisjunction of the chromosomes during meiosis. For reasons not yet understood, the frequency of this phenomenon increases with maternal age. Estimates are that at age 35 the risk of a liveborn child with Down Syndrome is one in 385, at age 40 the risk is one in 106, and at age 45 the risk is one in 30. However, since there are more births of children to young women, most children with Down syndrome are born to mothers younger than age 35.

Most of the genes that cause the symptoms of Down syndrome appear to be located on the long arm of chromosome 21. Sometimes a piece of a chromosome can wander on to another chromosome, a process known as a *translocation*. If a wandering piece of the long arm of chromosome 21 is present in addition to two normal copies of chromosome 21, there can be clinical symptoms of Down syndrome in a person with the normal number of chromosomes. About 3 percent of Down syndrome cases are due to a translocation. Three quarters of these translocations occur spontaneously. A quarter of the translocations are genetically passed down in families.

Living with the Condition

The prognosis for children with Down syndrome has markedly improved in recent decades. Part of this improvement is due to the norm of living at home as opposed to institutionalization. Another part is proper health care supervision, for which the American Academy of Pediatrics has guidelines.[2]

Once the diagnosis is made, people with this condition need to be followed by a number of specialists, both as children and as adults. Since half of all infants with Down syndrome are born with a congenital heart defect, a cardiologist should always be consulted. These heart defects are often diagnosed prenatally and in many cases do not require any treatment. On the other hand, some require various degrees of surgical intervention. The frequency of follow-up will depend on the particular heart issues that are found.

Due to the structure of their skulls, individuals with this condition are more likely to have ear infections and fluid in their ears that can affect hearing. Hearing loss based on reduced nerve function (sensorineural hearing loss) often occurs later in life but may start as early as age six. Therefore, hearing should be monitored in those with this condition. At a later age, hearing aids may be needed. People with Down syndrome also have a higher incidence of temporary cessation of breathing during sleep

(sleep apnea). For all these complaints, follow-up by an ear, nose, and throat specialist is important.

Infants with this condition tend to have hypotonia (low muscle tone), which can make feeding more challenging. With some initial guidance, most infants can be breastfed successfully. However, in some cases feeding therapy aimed at improving the ability to suck and swallow, or even the placement of a temporary feeding tube, may be required. Muscle tone generally improves with age.

Children with Down syndrome have specific dental conditions. Therefore, follow-up by a dentist familiar with their care is important.

Those with Down syndrome are at a higher risk of leukemia than those without the condition. Therefore, symptoms suggestive of this disease (bruising, pallor, enlarged lymph nodes) need to be evaluated. On the other hand, they have a lower than average risk of solid tumors; therefore, the overall risk of cancer is not increased.

Individuals with Down syndrome tend to be short. There are specific growth charts for such children available. Monitoring of growth is important, because those with this condition are at risk of developing thyroid dysfunction, which can itself impede growth. Periodic testing of thyroid function is also recommended. People with the condition are also at higher risk for celiac disease (sensitivity to gluten).

Individuals with Down syndrome tend to have instability of the joint that attaches the skull to the spine. Evaluation for this condition needs to be undertaken before they participate in certain sports.

Infants will be delayed in reaching developmental milestones. However, early intervention with physical, occupational, and speech therapy has been shown to improve the level of function.

In older children and adults, mental retardation is generally in the mild to moderate range. Many children with this condition can be accommodated in the regular school system. Many adults live completely independently and are employed. Others live independently in assisted-living situations.

Sources

H. Chen, Down Syndrome. eMedicine Pediatrics.
http://emedicine.medscape.com/article/943216

Suggested Reading
Down Syndrome. Genetics Home Reference.
http://ghr.nlm.nih.gov/condition/down-syndrome
The website www.ds-health.com contains a collection of essays on health-related issues of Down syndrome, compiled by a pediatrician who is also the father of a son with the condition.
The website www.down-syndrome-facts-and-fiction.com is a collection put together by the mother of a child with Down syndrome.

Support Organizations
The National Down Syndrome Society
666 Broadway, 8th Floor
New York, NY 10012-2317
Phone: (212) 460-9330 or (800) 221-4602
Fax: (212) 979-2873
Email: info@ndss.org
National Down Syndrome Congress
1370 Center Drive, Suite 102
Atlanta, GA 30338
Phone: (770) 604-9500 or (800) 232-NDSC
Email: info@ndscenter.org
National Association for Down Syndrome
PO Box 206
Wilmette, IL 60091
Phone: (630) 325-9112
The Arc
The Arc of the United States
1010 Wayne Avenue, Suite 650
Silver Spring, MD 20910
Phone: (301) 565-3842

---

1. See the section on genetic testing for more information on commonly used tests for detection.
2. AAP Committee on Genetics, Policy Statement: Health Supervision for Children with Down Syndrome. *Pediatrics* 2001; 107:442–49. Reaffirmed May 2007.

Fragile X Syndrome

Summary

Fragile X syndrome consists of varying degrees of mental retardation and abnormal (autistic-like) behavior or hyperactivity. It is the second most common cause of mental retardation.[1] Beginning in adolescence, boys affected with the condition tend to have a distinctive physical appearance. They are prone to scoliosis (curvature of the spine), mitral valve prolapse (having the leaves of one of the heart valves close in an abnormal fashion), and strabismus (cross eye). They also commonly experience gastroesophageal reflux and ear infections. Some have a seizure disorder as well.

The abnormality is found on the X chromosome. Because females have two X chromosomes, one of which is turned off while the other expresses its genetic makeup, there is a 50 percent chance that a girl who has inherited an affected chromosome will have the condition. The degree of retardation tends to be less severe in females. Therefore, most cases of fragile X, and certainly the more severe cases, appear in males.

Historical Background

In 1943 James P. Martin and Julia Bell reported a family with multiple male members with mental retardation. Therefore, this condition is at times called *Martin Bell syndrome.*

Diagnosis of Condition

Fragile X is one of the conditions considered in patients with delayed speech, autistic types of behaviors (poor eye contact, hand biting, hand flapping), or mental retardation. It will be suspected faster in families with a history of multiple male relatives with mental retardation. However, since it is one of the most common causes of mental retardation, a search for Fragile X is generally part of a diagnostic workup for developmental delay.[2] In adolescence, affected males tend to develop a characteristic facial appearance that includes a long thin face with prominent ears, forehead, and jaw. The testicles of adult males are large. The disease is confirmed by DNA testing.

Genetic Cause

The condition is almost always associated with too many repeats of CGG (cystine, guanine, guanine) in the FMR 1 gene on the distal end of the long arm of the X chromosome. Furthermore, the expanded gene generally has methyl groups attached to it. People with the full mutation (more than 200 repeats), especially if the repeated sections are methylated, cannot produce a functioning fragile X mental retardation protein, a protein found in nerve cells. Lack of functioning protein leads to abnormal connections between nerve cells.

A somewhat elevated number of repeats (55–200 repeats) is known as a *premutation*.[3] About one-third of older men and about 5 percent of older women with a premutation will have a syndrome called *fragile X associated tremor/ataxia syndrome* (FXTAS) and have problems with balance and signs of neurodegeneration. About 25 percent of women with a premutation will experience premature ovarian failure. Levels of 41–60 repeats are sometimes defined as being in an intermediate or gray zone. People with this level are unaffected, but there may be a higher chance of a premutation or full mutation developing in a later generation.

Heredity

The disease is inherited in an X linked manner. Because of the variable penetration and varying levels of severity, the exact carrier frequency is not known. However, it is estimated to be approximately one in 130–250 females and one in 250–800 males. In an Israeli-based study, the number of women carrying a gene with more than 54 CGG repeats was 1:113.[4] Other Israeli studies found a carrier frequency of 1:150. A higher frequency is found in Jews of Tunisian origin, especially those from the island of Djerba.

Males with a premutation pass this on to their daughters. They do not pass it on to their sons, since their sons receive the Y chromosome from them rather than the X. Females with a premutation are usually unaffected, although about one-third are mildly affected. The number of CGG triples can increase from generation to generation, although not in a predictable manner. The number of repeats is directly proportional to the chance of an offspring's being affected.

Living with the Condition

The American Academy of Pediatrics has published guidelines for the health supervision of those with this condition.[5] They need educational assistance in order to reach their maximum potential. Children who grow up in high-functioning homes and receive appropriate educational services are most likely to have higher intellectual achievement and improved behavior. Therefore, children suspected or known to have the condition should be referred for early multidisciplinary evaluation (speech, physical and occupational therapy) and for early intervention programs geared to their individual needs.

Dealing with the behavioral issues can be difficult. Family counseling can help teach behavior modification strategies. The hyperactivity and attention deficit can be moderated with the use of stimulants such as methylphenidate or amphetamines. Clonidine can be used as well in young children, especially those with sleep disorders. Medication may be used for management of seizures or reflux as well.

Sources
R. A. Sauland, J. C. Tarletone, FMR1-Related Disorders. GeneReviews. http://www.ncbi.nlm.nih.gov/books/NBK1384/
J. A. Jewell. Fragile X Syndrome. eMedicine Pediatrics. http://emedicine/medscape/com/article/943776-overview
R. J. Hagerman, E. Berry-Kravis, W. E. Kaufmann, et al., Advances in the Treatment of Fragile X Syndrome. *Pediatrics* 2009; 123: 378–90.
J. Zlotogara, Mendelian Disorders Among Jews. www.health.gov.il/Download/pages/book_jews7.pdf

Suggested Reading
Fragile X Syndrome. Genetics Home Reference. http://ghr.nlm.nih.gov/condition/fragile-x-syndrome.

Support Organizations
FRAXA Research Foundation
45 Pleasant Street
Newburyport, MA 09150
Phone: (978) 462-1866
Fax: (978) 463-9985
Email: info@fraxa.org
Internet: www.fraxa.org
Conquer Fragile X Foundation
Email: mail@cfxf.org
Internet: www.conquerfragilex.org
Living with Fragile X
Email: info@livingwithfragilex.com

The National Fragile X Foundation
PO Box 37
Walnut Creek, CA 94597
Phone: (800) 688-8765
Fax: (925) 938-9315
Email: natlfx@FragileX.org
Internet: www.FragileX.org

1. Trisomy 21, or Down syndrome, is the first.
2. J. B. Moeschler, M. Shevell, and the AAP Committee on Genetics. Clinical genetic evaluation of the child with mental retardation or developmental delays. *Pediatrics* 2006; 117: 2304–16.
3. There is some debate as to the exact cutoffs of each category.
4. H. Toledano-Aldehef, L. Baseel-Vanagiate, N. Magal, et al., Fragile-X carrier screening and the prevalence of premutation and full mutation carriers in Israel. *Am J Hum Genetic* 2001; 69:351–60.
5. AAP Committee on Genetics, Policy Statement: Health Supervision for Children with Fragile X Syndrome. *Pediatrics* 1996; 98:297–300. Reaffirmed May 2007.

Spinal Muscle Atrophy

Summary

Spinal Muscle Atrophy (SMA) is a group of disorders in which there is degeneration of the motor nerve cells in the spinal cord. This degeneration leads to progressive muscle weakness and paralysis. The form of SMA that involves the proximal muscles (those of the torso and upper part of the arms and legs) has three types, differentiated according to onset and severity. Type I, also known as *Werdnig Hoffman disease*, is characterized by severe muscle weakness and low muscle tone (*hypotonia*) from birth or within the first three months of life. Those with this condition generally die from respiratory failure by age two. In type II the degeneration begins later and the weakness is less. Children with this type generally learn to sit, although not to walk. They generally live to approximately four years. Type III SMA (*Kugelberg Welander disease*) is the mildest form. Onset begins in infancy or childhood. The children learn to walk unaided and generally live until the teenage years.

Sixty percent of cases of SMA are type I. It is the most common lethal genetic disease in the general population.

Historical Background

In 1891 Dr. Guido Werdnig, an Austrian neurologist, and Dr. Johann Hoffman, a German neurologist, independently reported an infantile form of muscular dystrophy. SMA I thus bears their names. In 1956 Drs. Erik Kugelberg and Lisa Welander, Swedish neurologists, described the less severe form of SMA, and thus type III bears their names.

Diagnosis of Condition

Type I SMA is one of the conditions suspected when a child has hypotonia at birth. Other forms are suspected in children with hypotonia and developmental delay. Finding a mutation in the SMA1 gene confirms the condition.

Screening for this condition is now part of many prenatal genetic panels. However, while all agree that screening in affected families makes sense, there is debate as to whether the general public should be screened for this condition.[1] The American College of Medical Geneticists feels that this testing should be offered to all couples of all ethnic groups.[2] The American College of Obstetricians and Gynecologists (ACOG)

Committee on Genetics feels that preconception and prenatal screening for SMA is not recommended in the general population at this time.[3]

Genetic Cause

All three forms of SMA are associated with mutations in the SMA1 gene. However, expression of the condition can be modified by the SMA2 gene. More copies of the SMA2 gene seem to lead to a milder course of the disease. These two genes are found next to each other on the long arm of chromosome 5.

Heredity

The condition is inherited in an autosomal recessive manner. The carrier frequency among Ashkenazi Jews (1:46) is slightly lower than that in the general Caucasian population (1:37).[4]

Living with the Condition

Intellectual development is normal. However, the hypotonia can prevent affected children from reaching developmental milestones.

Care for type I is mostly supportive. Insertion of a gastrostomy (feeding) tube may prevent pneumonia due to aspiration. However, the progressive hypotonia generally leads to breathing difficulties and eventual death.

Children with types II and III can benefit from physical therapy to maintain muscle tone as long as possible, as well as assistance through the use of adaptive equipment.

Because this condition, especially type 1, has a known fatal outcome, it is likely to raise questions regarding how much intervention to do for prolonging life. This is a question in which a halachic authority should be involved at an early stage. Halachic considerations should be part of individual decisions made.[5]

Sources

T. W. Prior and B. S. Russman, Spinal Muscle Atrophy. GeneReviews. http://www.ncbi.nlm.nih.gov/books/NBK1352/
B. Tsao and C. Armon. eMedicine Neurology. http://emedicine.medscape.com/article/1181436-overview

Suggested Reading

Spinal Muscle Atrophy. Genetics Home Reference. http://ghr.nlm.nih.gov/condition/spinal-muscular-atrophy

Support Organizations
Families of Spinal Muscle Atrophy
925 Busse Road
Elk Grove Village, IL 60007
Phone: (800) 866-1762
Email: info@fsma
Internet: www.fsma.org

---

1. The primary cause of the debate is whether there are enough resources to provide sufficient counseling to the public at large to justify mass screening for this condition.

2. Prior, T.W.; for the Professional Practice and Guidelines Committee. Carrier screening for spinal muscular atrophy. *Genetics in Medicine* 2008; 10:1–3.

3. Spinal muscular atrophy, ACOG Committee Opinion No. 432, American College of Obstetricians and Gynecologists. *Obstet Gynecol* 2009; 113:1194–96.

4. B. C. Hendrickson, C. Donohoe, V. R. Akmaev, et al., Differences in SMN1 allele frequencies among ethnic groups in North America. *J. Med. Genet.* published online July 21, 2009. Available at http://jmg.bmj.com/content/46/9/641. Accessed November 13, 2010.

5. See chapter on Death of a Child.

Turner Syndrome

Summary

Turner syndrome is a condition affecting girls, in which there is short stature and lack of sexual development.

Girls with Turner syndrome may be born with a number of clinical findings. Some have extra skin on the neck, a condition known as *webbing*. They may have swollen hands and feet and unusually shaped nails. Some have none of these findings. They grow slowly and will be short for their age.

Children with this condition may have one of a number of congenital heart defects.[1] Unless specifically looked for, these defects may not be noticed until later in life. Those with the condition are at higher risk of having high blood pressure. The aorta, the large artery that brings blood from the heart to the rest of the body, has a greater tendency than normal to burst.

Individuals with Turner syndrome have the external appearance of girls. Internally, most of them have normal female anatomy as well. However, the ovaries are likely to fail prematurely. Therefore, without treatment, most of those with this condition will not develop secondary sex characteristics, such as breasts, in adolescence, and they will be infertile. In the case of a mosaic (46XY,45X0), there is glandular tissue that more closely resembles testes. These gonads are at high risk of becoming cancerous and therefore are generally removed.

Historical Background

The syndrome is named after Dr. Henry Turner, who was among the first to describe its features in the 1930s. However, it was likely noted already in antiquity; see the section on disorders of sexual development.

Diagnosis of Condition

The condition is suspected when a female infant is born with swelling of the hands or feet, extra skin on the neck, and the characteristic heart lesions. It is suspected later in life in girls who are short for their age or do not show signs of puberty at the expected times. It is further suspected by finding high levels of follicular stimulating hormone (FSH). It can be confirmed by performing a karyotype—a test for the number of chromosomes found in a cell, generally done on white blood cells.

Genetic Cause
The condition occurs when a fetus loses all or part of one sex (X or Y) chromosome. This may affect all the cells or only some of them (the latter situation is known as *mosaicism*). Many pregnancies with Turner syndrome babies will end in spontaneous abortion. The rest produce infants born with the some or none of the clinical features of the condition

Heredity
This condition happens very early in pregnancy. It is *not* inherited from a parent.

Living with the Condition
Once the diagnosis is made, people with this condition need to be followed by a number of specialists, both as children and as adults. One is a cardiologist. The frequency of follow-up will depend on the particular heart issues that are found. It is important to continue to monitor for normal blood pressure and to treat high blood pressure if found.

An endocrinologist is an important specialist for those with this condition. Use of human growth factor has been shown to increase the growth of girls with Turner syndrome and is frequently used. With the approach of adolescence, estrogen is generally given to allow for development of a normal female appearance. Those with Turner syndrome are at high risk of developing autoimmune thyroiditis (inflammation of the thyroid caused by the body's reacting against itself) and needing thyroid hormone replacement.

Kidney abnormalities are not uncommon and should be searched for. Strabismus (cross eye) is more common and thus all girls with this condition should see an ophthalmologist at one year of age, in addition to routine screening.

Girls with this condition are more likely to have ear infections and fluid in their ears that can affect hearing, due to the structure of their skulls. Sensorineural hearing loss often occurs later in life but may start as early as age six. Therefore, hearing should be monitored in those with this condition. At a later age, hearing aids may be needed.

Lymphatic swelling may occur and can be treated. The National Lymphedema Network (www.lymphnet.org) can provide more information on the treatment of this symptom. Girls with this condition are at higher risk of developing dislocation of the hips, and/or curvature of the spine such as scoliosis and kyphosis. They are also at higher risk of developing celiac disease—sensitivity to gluten, a protein found in wheat. They should be tested for this condition (a blood test for specific antibodies) on an ongoing basis. If the condition is found, dietary treatment consisting of avoidance of gluten plus supervision by a gastroenterologist is needed.

Because of the premature ovarian failure, most girls with this condition will not be able to conceive without medical assistance. Artificial reproductive technology with donated eggs is a possibility (see chapter on Artificial Reproductive Technologies and Genetic Diseases). Pregnancy may increase the risk of rupture of the aorta and thus should be managed by a high-risk team.

Sources
A. Bondy and the Turner Syndrome Study Group, Clinical Practice Guideline.
Care of Girls and Women with Turner Syndrome: A Guideline of the Turner Syndrome Study Group. *The Journal of Clinical Endocrinology & Metabolism* 92:10–25.
A. C. Postellon and M. S. Daniel, Turner Syndrome. eMedicine.
http://emedicine/medscape/com/article/949681-overview

Suggested Reading
Turner Syndrome. Genetics Home Reference.
http://ghr.nlm.nih.gov/condition/turner-syndrome
Turner Syndrome. Human Growth Foundation.
http://www.hgfound.org/pub_turner.htm

Support Organizations
Turner Syndrome Society of the United States
11250 West Road, Suite G
Houston, TX 77065
Phone: (800) 365-9944
Fax: (832) 912-6446
Email: tssusadmin1@gmail.com
Internet: www.turnersyndrome.org
Turner Syndrome Foundation
Box 726
Holmdel, NJ 07733
Phone: (800) 594-4585
Internet: www.turnersyndromefoundation.org

The MAGIC Foundation—Corporate Office
6645 West North Avenue
Oak Park, IL 60302
Phone: (800) 362-4423
Internet: www.magicfoundation.org

---

1. Usually either aortic coarctation or an aortic valve with two flaps instead of three (bicuspid).

Disorders of Sexual Development

Mazal tov! It's a girl! Congratulations! It's a boy!

At times, making such a statement is not so simple. Some babies are born with external genitalia that do not fit clearly into what we are used to for either category. This phenomenon is often called *ambiguous genitalia*. There are a number of conditions that can lead to this situation.

Sexual Development

In order to better understand disorders of sexual development, it is important to understand how gender development generally takes place.

If one could look at an embryo up to the age of six weeks, one would not be able to tell what gender it would eventually become. Regardless of whether its sex chromosomes are XX or XY, the appearance at this point is identical. The embryo has two sex hormone producing glands (gonads) that can develop into either testes or ovaries. There is a proto-phallus, which can become a penis or clitoris, and labioscrotal folds, which can become labia or a scrotum. The embryo will also start to develop two sets of ducts. The *Wolffian ducts* develop into male structures and the *Mullerian ducts* develop into female structures.

Sexual differentiation takes place through the SRY gene, which is generally present on the Y chromosome. For this reason, most embryos that have a Y chromosome will develop into males. Embryos without a Y chromosome will generally develop into females. Rarely, the SRY gene can be misplaced onto another chromosome. Should this happen, an embryo that is XX will develop male structures. Furthermore, an embryo that is XXY, a condition called *Klinefelter syndrome*, will also develop male structures.

If the SRY gene is present, then the gonads will develop into the testes. The testes secrete *androgens* (male hormones), which cause the Wolffian ducts to develop into the male external genitalia. In the process of development, the proto-phallus develops into the penis, the labioscrotal folds join to become the scrotum, and the urethra lengthens. The testes also secrete *Mullerian-inhibiting substance* (MIS), which causes the Mullerian ducts not to develop further and to regress.

When the SRY gene is absent or not functional, the gonads will develop into ovaries. The Wolffian ducts regress and the Mullerian ducts develop into the internal female organs (uterus, fallopian tubes, and upper part of the vaginal canal). The proto-phallus becomes the clitoris, the labioscrotal folds remain divided, and the urethra remains short. For this reason, those who are XX, XO, or XXX will be born with female external genitalia.

Sometimes the Y chromosome is present but the body is unresponsive to the androgens that are produced. This condition is known as *androgen insensitivity syndrome*. If this insensitivity is complete, the external genitalia will be female, internal testes instead of ovaries, and no uterus. When there is partial insensitivity, there can be a variable appearance of the external genitalia.

At puberty, additional changes take place. If all parts of the body are working as expected, in a male, androgens from the adrenal glands and testes will lead to other masculinizing changes, known as *male secondary sex characteristics*, such as male-pattern pubic hair (diamond-shaped distribution), prominence of the Adam's apple, and deepening voice. If the testes are not functioning or there is a lack of response to the androgens, boys will not develop these signs. In a female, estrogen from the ovaries will lead to the development of breasts and female-pattern pubic hair (triangular-shaped-distribution). If the ovaries are not working, then these female secondary sex characteristics will not be present. For menstruation, one needs (1) functioning ovaries to produce the necessary hormones; (2) a functioning uterus to respond to the hormones with shedding of the lining; and (3) an open vaginal canal to allow the menstrual discharge to exit.

Understanding these stages of development helps one understand the findings in specific disorders of sexual development. Here are a number of examples:

1. Girls with Turner syndrome (XO) are born with external female genitalia, since they do not have a Y chromosome. However, because many of them will have early loss of ovarian function, without medical intervention they will not develop breasts or menstruation. As in all females, there is secretion of androgens from the adrenal glands. Without the estrogen to balance it out, this can lead to some voice deepening.

2. Girls with the severe forms of Congenital Adrenal Hyperplasia have XX (and no Y) chromosomes. For this reason, they develop female internal organs, but the enzyme blockages in the adrenal glands lead to overproduction of androgens. These androgens cause the proto-phallus and labioscrotal folds to follow the male pattern of development. Depending on the degree of blockage and thus the amount of overproduction, the result can range from a

prominent clitoris alone to fused labia and very prominent clitoris that can be mistaken for male external genitalia, and many steps along the continuum would appear both male and female.

3. Persons with complete androgen insensitivity develop all external female signs. While the Y chromosome is present and the internally located testes are producing testosterone, the receptors for this hormone are not functioning. Therefore, it is as if the testosterone were not there. Such children will be assumed to be girls and will likely be unaware of their condition unless they undergo a workup because of lack of menstruation.

4. Those with partial androgen insensitivity may develop external genitalia along the male/female spectrum depending on the degree of insensitivity. Internally they will have testes and no uterus.

5. Those with deficiency of the enzymes 5 alpha reductase and 17B hydroxysulfatase are XY but are born with external genitalia that more resemble female anatomy. With puberty they start to develop male-pattern pubic and axillary hair and muscle development and begin to feel like boys. This circumstance is due to the fact that they can produce testosterone but not 5 alpha dihydrotestosterone, which is needed for the genital development in utero but not for secondary sexual characteristics. The testosterone produced later in life can have some effect on the phallus, leading to phallic enlargement.

Disorders of Sexual Development in Traditional Jewish Sources

Disorders of sexual development existed at the time of the Talmud. The Talmud mentions several halachic concepts that refer to abnormal gender development. Trying to match them with modern-day diagnoses is not simple, but a number of hints can lead to some guesses.

One such term is an *eilonit*. The *mishna* in *Niddah* 5:9 says that a woman who has not developed pubic hair by the time she is known to be 20 years of age is considered an *eilonit*. Because an *eilonit* is infertile, and thus there was never the chance of her having children, neither levirite marriage (*yibbum*) nor the ceremony to release one from the levirite marriage (*chalitza*) needs to be performed should her husband die childless. Rashi explains the etymology of this word as coming from *eyal*—a male sheep, indicating that there are some masculine characteristics of one who has this condition. In his commentary on *Yevamot* 42b, he further points out that she develops neither breasts nor pubic hair. The signs that are described are reminiscent of Turner syndrome (see the section on that condition).

The *mishna* in *Yevamot* 8:6 mentions three terms related to conditions of unusual genitalia: the *saris chama*, the *androgynos,* and the *tumtum.* This *mishna* states that the wife of a *saris chama* who is a *kohen* is entitled to eat *terumah*, indicating that marriage to this *saris chama* is a fully valid marriage, despite the individual's lack of testes and thus inability to bear children. This fact needs to be pointed out, because in most cases marriage to a man whose testicles are absent (*patzua daka*) is forbidden by the Torah.[1] The Talmud (*Yevamot* 79b–80a) resolves the contradiction by pointing out that there are two categories of those with missing testicles. The biblical prohibition applies to the *saris adam*, one who has had the testicles surgically removed. It does not apply to the *saris chama*, defined in the Talmud as one who has never had testicles.[2] In context, however, he has other male sexual organs and thus can be married to a woman. The disorder of sexual development that bests fits this description is a deficiency of the enzymes 5 alpha reductase or 17B hydroxysulfatase. With these deficiencies, testes may not be noted at birth but secondary male sexual characteristics develop with puberty.[3]

The *androgynos*, from its meaning in Greek and from the contexts in which it is used in the Talmud, is one who has the signs of both male and female sexual development. This most likely refers to the medical situation generally called *ambiguous genitalia*,[4] which is caused by either partial androgen insensitivity or congenital adrenal hyperplasia.[5]

Tumtum is the most difficult talmudic condition for which to find a modern equivalent. It is understood in traditional sources[6] as one who does not have the external signs of either gender. In addition, the sources talk about removing some sort of covering and being able to determine the gender. There currently does not seem to be such a situation.

The halachic status of those with unclear genitalia has been a matter of halachic debate since the time of the Mishna. One possibility is that there is a clear gender identity. Another is that they fit into their own category. The third is that they are possibly (*safek*) male and possibly (*safek*) female and thus the manner in which they perform commandments has to take into considerations the obligations of both genders.[7] For example, a *brit milah* is performed, and the person may not shave with a razor and, if a *kohen*, may not have contact with the dead. All positive commandments, even those not incumbent upon women (e.g., *tefillin*), have to be observed.

In practice, it is the last opinion that holds sway. By most opinions, an *androgynos* can marry a woman and cannot marry a man. However, since the rules are complex, and marriage has significant halachic implications, an individual *psak* should be obtained from a prominent rabbi with experience in these laws.

Gender Assignment

Much of child raising depends on gender assignment. Even in places with equal co-education, there are generally some activities divided along gender lines (e.g., sports, Scout troops). At the very least, grammar requires the assignment of gender to be able to know whether to say *he* or *she*. Therefore, much thought needs to be given soon after birth as to what gender to assign the child.

Gender assignment also has significant halachic implications. For example, there are gender differences in ritual obligations (e.g., men are required to wear *tefillin*, women are not; men count toward the *minyan*, women do not) and personal status (e.g., to which gender to be married). Furthermore, dressing in the garments of the opposite gender is forbidden.[8]

The upbringing of children with disorders of sexual development is complex. An excellent handbook is available from the Consortium for the Management of Disorders of Gender Development. Because of the additional halachic implications involved, a rabbi who is familiar with this difficult area of *halacha* should be consulted as well.

Gender Assignment Surgery

In the past, gender assignment was made primarily on the basis of ease of reconstructing external genitalia, and surgery was performed in infancy to give the external appearance of the assigned gender.[9] This meant that the child has no input in the decision. A number of studies showed that a significant number of children felt that the surgery had significant impact on their sexual function and/or were not happy with the gender to which they were assigned. There are those who consider it unethical for parents to make this decision for their children.[10] The tendency today is to attempt to delay surgery until the child can have some say in the outcome.[11, 12]

For technical reasons, it is often easier to reconstruct female organs than male organs. For this reason, many individuals with ambiguous genitalia underwent reconstruction to form labia and vagina, had the testes removed, were given estrogens, and were raised as girls. The removal of the testes was to prevent male hormones from leading to male-pattern development in adolescence. Testes or undifferentiated gonads that remain internal are also at higher risk of turning cancerous.

This surgical approach, however, raises a number of halachic issues. First of all, if an *androgynos* had the obligations of a male, it would be easier to raise him as a male. Furthermore, as is discussed above under *saris adam*, removal of testes is a clear halachic prohibition. For this reason, Rav Avraham Sofer rules that this surgery should not be performed unless it is clear that the internal organs are in fact female. In practical terms, this would mean that those with virilized CAH would be allowed to undergo reconstructions but those with other disorders of sexual development would not.[13] Rav Eliezer Waldenberg discusses the rule of the *tumtum* and *androgynos* at length.[14] In his opinion, the most important deciding factor is the external visual appearance. Therefore, where the external appearance was clearly female (such as androgen insensitivity), any needed reconstruction would be allowed. The testes can be removed, in his opinion, because removal of the testes is not what would lead to infertility and thus does not fall under the prohibition of sterilization.[15] Rav Shlomo Zalman Auerbach also allows the removal of the testes, since they are at risk of becoming cancerous.[16]

In actual cases, decisions regarding surgery are complicated. Parents are best served by getting the input of many professionals, including mental health professionals with expertise in this area. Jewish parents should also be sure to include a rabbi familiar with this area of Jewish law in this team.

Support Organizations
Intersex Society of North America (ISNA)
979 Golf Course Drive, #282
Rohnert Park, CA 94928
Internet: www.isna.org
Androgen Insensitivity Syndrome Support Group (AISSG)
PO Box 2148
Duncan, OK 73534-2148
Internet: www.aissgusa.org
Androgen Insensitivity Syndrome Support Group UK
Internet: www.medhelp.org/www/ais
AISSG Australia
PO Box 1089, Altona Meadows
Victoria, Australia 3028

Phone/Fax: +61 3 9315 8809
Email: aissg@iprimus.com
Internet: www.vicnet.net.au/~aissg
Androgen Insensitivity Syndrome Support Group Canada (East)
#206, 115 The Esplanade
Toronto, Ont. M5E 1Y7 Canada
Email: sallie@ican.net (English)
Androgen Insensitivity Syndrome Support Group Canada (West)
#17, 3031 Williams Road
Richmond, BC V7E 1H9 Canada
Email: lesnick@shaw.ca
CARES Foundation
Congenital Adrenal Hyperplasia Education & Support
189 Main Street, 2nd Floor
Millburn, NJ 07041
Internet: www.caresfoundation.org
Hypospadias & Epispadias Association (HEA)
240 West 44th Street, Suite 1A
New York, NY 10036
Internet: www.heainfo.org
Klinefelter Syndrome and Associates
11 Keats Court
Coto de Caza, CA 92679
The Magic Foundation
6645 West North Avenue
Oak Park, IL 60302
Internet: www.magicfoundation.org
MRKH Organization
PO Box 301494
Jamaica Plain, MA 02130
Internet: www.mrkh.org
Turner Syndrome Society of the U.S.
14450 TC Jester, Suite 260
Houston, TX 77014
Internet: www.turner-syndrome-us.org
XY Turner
Box 5166
Laurel, MD 20726
Internet: www.xyxo.org

1. *Devarim* 23:2.

2. *Yevamot* 72b.

3. This connection has been developed further by J. H. Barth and M. Zemer. The Congenital Eunuch: a medical-halachic study. Available at http://www.jewish virtuallibrary.org/jsource/Judaism/Eunuch.pdf. Accessed October 6, 2010. This article analyzes a recorded historical halachic case related to this condition.

4. The terminology used in describing these conditions is very charged. Traditionally, the term was ambiguous genitalia. A more recent term is intersex, the term preferred by the support organizations of those who have these conditions. Some who have the condition object to the terminology "disorder." See http://www. medhelp.org/ais/21_overview.htm# for a further discussion of the difficulties of the terminology used from the point of view of those with this condition.

5. See A. Cohen, Tumtum and androgynous. *Journal of Halacha and Contemporary Society* 1999; 38. Available at www.daat.ac.il/DAAT/english/journal/cohen-1.htm.

6. Such as Rambam *Hilchot Ishut* 2:25.

7. Rambam *Hilchot Avoda Zara* 12:4.

8. *Devarim* 22.

9. AAP Committee on Genetics, Section on Endocrinology, Section on Urology. Evaluation of the Newborn with Developmental Anomalies of the External Genitalia. *Pediatrics* 2000; 106:138-42. This policy has now been replaced by A. Lee, C. P. Houk, S. F. Ahmed, et al., Consensus statement of management of intersex disorders. *Pediatrics* 2006; 118; 3488–500. This updated statement reads: "It is generally felt that surgery that is performed for cosmetic reasons in the first year of life relieves parental distress and improves attachments between the child and the parents; the systematic evidence for this belief is lacking."

10. For an in-depth discussion of the general ethics of this topic, see: H. G. Beh and M. Diamond, An Emerging Ethical and Medical Dilemma: Should Physicians Perform Sex Assignment on Infants with Ambiguous Genitalia? *Michigan Journal of Gender & Law*, Vol. 7 (1): 1–63, 2000. Available online at http://www.hawaii.edu/PCSS/biblio/articles/2000to2004/2000-emerging-ethical-dilemma.html.

11. W. G. Reiner, Sex assignment in the neonate with intersex or inadequate genitalia, *Arch Pediatr Adolesc Med* 1997; 151:1044–45.

M. Diamond and H. K. Sigmundson, Management of intersexuality: guidelines for dealing with persons with ambiguous genitalia, *Arch Pediatr Adolesc Med* 1997; 151:1046–50.

12. A full set of clinical treatment guidelines for physicians and a handbook for patients are available from the Consortium for the Treatment of Disorders of Sexual Development. This can be accessed online at www.dsdguidelines.org.

13. *Nishmat Avraham Even HaEzer* 44:3. Available online at http://www.med ethics.org.il/articles/NA2/NishmatAbraham.eh.44.asp. Rav Shlomo Zalman Auerbach is also quoted in this source as allowing such surgery.

14. *Ttitz Eliezer* 3:13.
15. *Ttitz Eliezer* 11:78
16. *Nishmat Avraham Even HaEzer* 5:5.

Predisposition to Diseases

At times, a genetic mutation does not lead directly to a disease, but rather predisposes one to diseases. This can occur through a number of mechanisms. With the increase in genetic knowledge, it is likely that the list of such mutations will continue to grow.

Familial Hypercholesterolemia

Having a high blood level of cholesterol is part of a process that can block arteries, including those leading to the heart. Therefore, high levels of cholesterol predispose one to heart attacks. Cholesterol, however, is not the only factor involved in bringing about heart attacks. Therefore, a genetic condition that causes high cholesterol is an example of a genetic predisposition, not a direct genetic disease.

Jews of Lithuanian ancestry have a high carrier rate (1:67 as opposed to 1:500 in the general population) of a mutation in the gene for the LDL receptor protein, which is located on the short arm of chromosome 19.[1] Those who have one copy of this gene have elevated levels of cholesterol from birth. However, they do not show symptoms of cholesterol build-up (known as *xanthomas*, yellow growths) until about age 20. They are at a higher risk for heart attacks. Those who have two copies of the gene develop extremely high levels of cholesterol in infancy and, unless treated aggressively, die of heart attacks by age 30.

This gene provides an interesting marker as to the migration of Jews from Lithuania. A preponderance of the mutation is found in South Africa, in Israel and in St. Petersburg.[2]

Sources

E. Citkowitz, Familial Hypercholesterolemia. eMedicine. http://emedicine. medscape.com/article/121298-overview

V. Meiner, D. Landsberger, N. Berkman, et al., A Common Lithuanian Mutation Causing Familial Hypercholesterolemia in Ashkenazi Jews. *Am. J. Hum. Genet.* 1991; 49:443–449.

Cancer Predisposition

Development of cancer is also the result of a process. Cells are meant to reproduce themselves. However, they are meant to do so under a system of controls. Cancer can result when the control system malfunctions. Certain diseases that have other symptoms predispose those who have them to having cancer. Two examples discussed in the Genetic Diseases section are Bloom syndrome and ataxia-telangiectasia. Other genetic mutations do not have outward manifestations but increase the chances of developing cancer. Three such mutations linked to Jews, primarily those of Ashkenazi Jewish descent, are discussed here.

BRCA1

In 1994, mutations of a gene on the long arm of chromosome 17 were found in a high percentage of families that had multiple cases of breast and/or ovarian cancer, especially cancers that occurred at a relatively young age. This gene is now called BRCA1, named for its association with an increased rate of breast cancer. Since that time, over 800 mutations have been found in this particular gene. Two specific mutations have been found to occur frequently among those of Ashkenazi Jewish descent. One, the 185delAG mutation, is found in approximately 1 percent of the Ashkenazi Jewish population. The second mutation linked to this ethnic group is the 5382insC mutation. This mutation is found in approximately 1.5 percent of individuals of Ashkenazi Jewish descent.

The BRCA1 gene codes for the *breast cancer susceptibility type 1* protein. This protein has numerous roles in the nucleus of the cell, including repairing damage to DNA. "Wear and tear" of the DNA is an ongoing process; the body is usually able to repair this damage and no harm occurs. However, it is believed that the incorrectly coded protein's inability to repair the DNA can lead to the abnormal proliferation of cells known as cancer. Due to its presumed role in preventing the abnormal cell growth, BRCA1 is considered a "tumor suppressor gene."

BRCA2

Also in 1994, another breast cancer-associated gene was discovered on the long arm of chromosome 13. This bears the name of BRCA2. It codes for the *breast cancer susceptibility type 2* protein, which is also found in the nucleus. This protein regulates the protein produced by the RAD51 gene, whose role is to repair DNA. This helps explain why it is associated with increased incidence of cancer. While BRCA2 is also a breast cancer-associated gene, those with mutations in the BRCA2 have a higher incidence of ovarian cancer compared to those with mutations in the BRCA1 gene.

The mutation that is associated with those of Ashkenazi Jewish descent is the 6174delT mutation. The frequency is approximately 1.5 percent in this population.

Both the BRCA1 and BRCA2 genes are inherited in an autosomal dominant manner. One only needs a mutation on one copy of the gene to be at higher risk. This one mutation can be inherited either from the father or the mother.

Having the mutation increases the possibility of developing breast cancer (even in men) or ovarian cancer. There may be increased risk of pancreatic cancer as well. Men with this gene are at higher risk of prostate cancer. Some studies have found an association with colon cancer, but others have not. With the BRCA2 gene, there seems to be elevation in the rate of cancer in additional systems, such as the gastrointestinal system and the skin.

Mutations in these genes have now been found in Jews of non-Ashkenazi descent as well. The Tyr978X BRCA1 mutation was detected in 1 percent of the average-risk Jewish Iraqi population and in 1.7 percent of high-risk Jewish non-Ashkenazi individuals.[3] A recent study has identified two mutations: p.A1708E in BRCA1 and c.67 + 1G > A (IVS2 + 1G > A) in BRCA2 in Jews whose families originated from the Iberian peninsula. In the high-risk families tested, the frequency of the two mutations was 26–31 percent.[4]

However, it is apparent that the picture is still unclear. Due to incomplete penetrance, not every person who has the gene will develop cancer over their lifetime. The cumulative risk of developing breast cancer before age 70 is approximately 85 percent for those with these mutations, as opposed to a cumulative risk of 12.5 percent in those without these mutations.

Furthermore, not every mutation in the gene has the same effect; some mutations may not cause disease at all. Those who possess a mutation in the gene *and* belong to a family with a high incidence of early onset breast and/or ovarian cancer seem to be at higher risk than those who have the mutation but not the family history. This leads to a great deal of confusion as to if and when to test for the mutation. The research on these genes is relatively recent and is ongoing. This chapter will soon be out of date, and thus it is important to consult with a specialist who keeps up with the field before attempting to make actual decisions.

While any individual medical decision should be discussed with one's own physician, the following are some important issues to consider when making decisions about testing. A key point to consider before doing any medical test is what one will do with this information. If it will change medical treatment, that is a reason to consider doing a test. Women who have a BRCA gene mutation and a family history of breast cancer are generally advised to have more frequent screening for breast cancer (such as mammograms, breast self-examination, and even MRIs). These changes in monitoring schedule are an example of how doing the test will make a difference.

There are studies that seem to indicate that breast cancer in those with the BRCA mutation is less likely to recur if even small tumors are treated with chemotherapy and not just removal of the lump. Those with the BRCA2 mutation with ovarian cancer seem to respond better when treated by protocols that contain platinum. Therefore, women who themselves have breast or ovarian cancer should consider doing this test, as it might change the way they are treated. Due to the high frequency of this mutation in the Ashkenazi Jewish population, those who have cancer and are from this ethnic group are generally strongly encouraged to have this test.

On the other hand, there are potential risks with testing for something that is only a prediction, not a diagnosis. The stress of knowing that one is at high risk of developing cancer is hard for some people to deal with. For others, the knowledge of having the predisposition gives them a sense of empowerment as they can do something about it. For some, the knowledge is more than they can handle. Therefore, while those with a family history but no current disease should certainly consider testing, the decision should be thought through carefully. The final decision whether or not to test needs to be an individual one.

In addition to the universal concerns about the impact on the individual and the family, the dilemma of whether to share results with relatives is also a halachic concern. *Not* notifying family members may be a violation of *lo ta'amod al dam re'echa* (the injunction not to stand idly by the blood of your fellow person; *Leviticus* 19:16). Sharing the information could be a fulfillment of the commandment to save lives. The need to inform, however, needs to be balanced against the woman's own need for privacy. Sharing the information also has sociologic concerns. Sharing the information too widely in a close-knit community could affect the willing-ness of others in the community to marry someone known to carry the mutation, or to marry into the family at all.

Another halachic concern is that the management of BRCA1 and BRCA2 carriers involves consideration of oopherectomy (surgical remov-al of the ovaries), which is a form of sterilization. Sterilization for women is a rabbinic prohibition.[5] While all halachic authorities would allow this when the woman's life is clearly endangered by the presence of ovaries, in cases where there is not yet clear consensus on the treatment, the halachic prohibition has to at least be considered.[6]

APC

In 1997, it was discovered that possessing a mutation in the adeno-matous polyposis coli (APC) gene on chromosome 5 was associated with having cancer of the colon or rectum (CRC). This gene codes for a protein that is involved in the suppression of tumors. A particular mutation, known as I1307K,[7] was carried by 28 percent of Jewish patients with colorectal cancer and with a family history of such cancer, but only found in 6.1 per-cent of unselected Ashkenazi Jewish individuals. Additional studies have confirmed this association in the Ashkenazi Jewish population but not in other ethnic groups nor in Ashkenazi Jews with other forms of cancer. Possession of this mutation seems to raise the risk of cancer by 10–20 per-cent above the baseline risk of approximately 7percent. Some reports have suggested that those with this mutation are more likely to have an earlier onset of their cancer.

In this condition as well, having the mutation does not mean having the cancer. It simply means a higher risk. Therefore, those known to carry the mutation would need to be screened for this cancer with tests such as colonoscopy at more frequent intervals than the general population. The correct frequency needs to be determined for the individual based on a number of factors (e.g., age, family history), including knowledge of hav-ing the mutation. Here too, the impact of the information on the rest of the family should be considered as well.

Sources
N. Petrucelli, M. B. Daly, G. L. Feldman *BRCA1* and *BRCA2* Heredi-tary Breast and Ovarian Cancer. www.ncbi.nlm.nih.gov/bookshelf/br.fcgi?book=gene&part=brca1

S. Syngal, D. Schrag, M. Falchuk, et al. Phenotypic Characteristics Associated With the *APC* Gene I1307K Mutation in Ashkenazi Jewish Patients With Colorectal Polyps. *JAMA* 2000; 284:857–860.

Support Organizations
As cancer is a common condition, there are multiple support organizations for cancer. The following are nationwide resources that can be used to find local groups.

Breast Cancer
Susan G. Komen for the Cure
http://ww5.komen.org
Sharsheret (particularly for young Jewish women facing breast cancer)
http://www.sharsheret.org

All Cancers
American Cancer Society
www.cancer.org
Association of Cancer Online Resources
http://www.acor.org/index.html

There are other conditions where it appears that certain ethnic groups have a greater prevalence of the condition. One such example is Crohn disease.

Crohn's Disease
Crohn's disease is a disease of inflammation of the bowel. It and ulcerative colitis are often linked together as inflammatory bowel disease (IBD). Crohn's disease generally manifests as abdominal pain, blood in stool, and diarrhea. In children it can also cause poor growth and malnutrition. Other symptoms, such as fevers and joint pains, can occur as well. It has been known for a long time that Ashkenazi Jews are over twice as likely to suffer from Crohn's disease and more likely to have a family history of the disease.

Crohn's is an example of a multifactorial disease. There seem to be genetic, environmental, and immunological components that contribute to the likelihood of a person having the disease. Therefore, it is not surprising that no one gene has been found to be associated with this condition. Similarly, there is no one mutation that is found in Ashkenazi Jews who have this condition. However, recent studies have begun to find some variants that are more common in Jews of Ashkenazi origin, which may explain some of the increased predilection in this community.

One of the genes associated with Crohn's is CARD15,[8] found on the long arm of chromosome 16.[9] In a study comparing Ashkenazi and non-Ashkenazi Jewish families with Crohn's disease to non-Jews of European ancestry with Crohn's,[10] the mutations of this gene were found to be the same in Jews as in non-Jews.[11] However, the percentage of people having at least one of these mutations was highest in Jews of central European ancestry. The incidence was also highest in those with a family history of Crohn's rather than an isolated case. In addition, a variant that had not been reported previously (N852S) was found only in those of Ashkenazi descent. Another study found variants associated with Crohn's disease specifically in Ashkenazi Jews on the short arm of chromosome 1 and the long arm of chromosome 3.[12] Yet another new variant was discovered in this study as well, although not specific to Jews.

Sources
A. B. Grossman, P. Mamula. Crohn Disease. eMedicine Pediatrics.
http://emedicine.medscape.com/article/928288-overview
G. Y. Wu, M. L. Coash, S. Nachimuthu. Crohn Disease. eMedicine Gastroenterology.
http://emedicine.medscape.com/article/172940-overview

Support Organizations
Crohn's and Colitis Foundation of America
386 Park Avenue South
New York, NY 10016-8804
Phone: (800) 932-2423
Fax (212) 779-4098
Internet: www.ccfa.org
Intestinal Disease Foundation
1323 Forbes Avenue
Suite 200
Pittsburgh, PA 15219
Phone: (412) 261-5888

The National Digestive Diseases Information Clearinghouse
2 Information Way
Bethesda, MD 20892
Phone: (301) 654-3810
Internet: www.niddk.nih.gov
The Pediatric Crohn's and Colitis Association
PO Box 18
Newton, MA 02168-0002
Phone: (617) 290-0902
Reach Out for Youth With Ileitis and Colitis
15 Chemung Place
Jericho, NY 11753
Phone: (516) 822-8010
Fax: (516) 822-8885
Crohn's and Colitis Foundation of Canada
21 St. Clair Avenue East
Suite 301
Toronto, Ontario M4T 1L9
Phone: (800) 387-1479
Internet: www.ccfc.ca/site.html
NACC: National Association for Colitis and Crohn's Disease
PO Box 205
St. Albans, Herts, AL1 1AB
01727-844296
Internet: www.nacc.org.uk

Over time, more and more diseases are likely to be proved to have at least a partial genetic basis. As this happens the list of diseases with links to Jewish descent is likely to grow. Diabetes, a disease resulting from inadequate function of insulin in controlling blood sugar, is likely to be next. A recent study has found that interactions between genes increased the risk of development of adult-onset diabetes.[13] Once again, there is room to be humble, as it is clear that there is much more to discover.

---

1. The specific mutation is a deletion of the amino acid glycine at position 167 of the protein.
2. M. Mandelshtam, K. Chakir, S. Shevtsov, et al. Prevalence of Lithuanian mutation among St. Petersburg Jews with familial hypercholesterolemia. *Hum Mutat.* 1998; 12(4): 255–8.

3. R. Shiri-Sverdlov, R. Gershoni-Baruch, G. Ichezkel-Hirsch et al. The Tyr978X BRCA1 Mutation in Non-Ashkenazi Jews: Occurrence in High-Risk Families, General Population and Unselected Ovarian Cancer Patients. *Community Genet* 2001; 4:50–55.

4. M. Sagi, A. Eilat, L. Ben Avi, et al. BRCA1/2 founder mutations in Jews of Sephardic origin. *Familial Cancer* epublished ahead of print, November 10, 2010.

5. *Shulchan Aruch Even HaEzer* 5:11.

6. P. Mor, K. Oberle. Ethical issues related to BRCA gene testing in orthodox Jewish women. *Nursing Ethics* 2008; 15:514–22. (This article contains a more comprehensive review of these issues using the example of a case study.)

7. An isoleucine-to-lysine variant at codon 1307 of the APC gene.

8. Also know as NOD2.

9. H.H. Fidder, S. Olschwang, B. Avidan, et al. Association between mutations in the CARD15 (NOD2) gene and Crohn's disease in Israeli Jewish patients. *Am J Med Genet A* 2003; 121A: 240–4.

10. T. Tukel, A. Shalata, D. Present, et al. Crohn Disease: Frequency and nature of CARD15 mutations in Ashkenazi and Sephardi/Oriental Jewish families. *Am J Hum Genet* 2004; 74: 623–636.

11. R702W, G908R, and L1007fs.

12. Y. Y. Shugart, M. S. Silverberg, R. H. Duerr, et al. An SNP linkage scan identifies significant Crohn's disease loci on chromosomes 13q13.3 and, in Jewish families, on 1p35.2 and 3q29. *Genes Immun* 2008; 9:161–7.

13. R. J. Neuman, J. Wasson, G. Atzmon, et al. Gene-gene interactions lead to higher risk for development of type 2 diabetes in an Ashkenazi Jewish population. *PLoS One* 2010; 5:e9903.

Section III:

Living With Genetic Diseases

Introduction

Genetic diseases happen to people. Therefore, it would not be proper to discuss the diseases without discussion of their impact on those affected by them, as well as their families. The previous section of the book focused on issues specific to each condition. The goal of this section is to address topics that many of these conditions have in common.

One has to be cognizant of the fact that people have feelings and different people may feel differently about the same situation. Finding the words to discuss the impact of genetic diseases is not easy. Some people find certain terminology to be offensive, while other people find the opposite to be offensive. For example, some people who do not have typical hearing prefer to be referred to as deaf and be viewed as part of the deaf culture.[1] Others prefer to be called hearing impaired and yet others hard of hearing.[1] Therefore, it should be pointed out at the outset that there is no intent to insult. An assortment of terminology is used with the clear realization that, unfortunately, at least someone will find a term troublesome.

The first two chapters in this section ("A Special Kind of Parenthood" and "The Disabled Among Us") are based on information derived primarily from parents and those in the field of rehabilitation. The next chapter is written by two specialists in the field of developmental disabilities. As will be seen, there can be different viewpoints on similar situations. The hope is that people will use those parts of these sections that they find helpful and realize that sections that do not seem to fit their experience may be helpful to someone else.

The next chapter summarizes halachic issues related to the kind of physical and mental disabilities that can be secondary to a number of the genetic diseases discussed here. Individual books could likely be written on each section, which is beyond the scope of this book. However, it is hoped that this chapter will at least increase awareness of the types of issues involved.

The final chapter was probably the hardest to write. Dealing with the death of a child is a heart-wrenching experience for all, including physicians. Nevertheless, a book that is attempting to show that genetic diseases are realities that families live with and not just academic discussions would not be complete without it.

As there is a principle in Judaism to end on a positive note,[2] we will conclude with some Torah-based thoughts.

---

1. See also the discussions about terminology in the section "Disorders of Sexual Development."
2. That is why some earlier verses are repeated at the end of certain books (such as *Eichah*).

A Special Kind of Parenthood

Raising any child is challenging.[1] Raising a child with special needs is all the more so. The goal of this section is to share what I have learned as a pediatrician (and parent) over the years as to how to approach this challenge. My personal experience was supplemented by a number of interviews with parents raising children with genetic conditions as well as with other professionals who work with special children.

A key role of a parent is to be your child's advocate. This is true for all children but all the more so for children with difficulties, be they mental, physical, or emotional. Following is a list of things one can do to fulfill this crucial role in the life of your special child.

Get as Much Information as You Can

Use reliable sources on the internet. For each condition discussed in this book we have provided at least one resource as a starting point for more information. The more you understand about what is known about your child's condition, the better positioned you are to help him or her reach maximum potential. Balance your research with the help of trained professionals. If there is information that you don't understand, make sure to ask. Your family pediatrician is likely to be happy to help make sense of all you are reading. Remember the dictum of Hillel in *Pirkei Avot:*[2] "*Lo habayshan lomed*—one who is embarrassed does not learn."

Here are some additional resources that cover a variety of conditions. They are useful for the conditions covered in this book as well as many others:

Madison's Foundation (www.madisonsfoundation.org) houses the **m-Power Rare Disease Database**. This database of explanations of rare diseases was written by medical professionals at UCLA in a way that can be understood by those who are not medical professionals. Children's Rare Disease Network (www.crdnetwork.org) has multidisease information available as well. For those living in the United Kingdom, a key resource is the National Information Center for Metabolic Diseases, known as CLIMB (Children Living with Metabolic Diseases, www.climb.org.uk).[3]

Remember, however, that all people, even people with special needs, are unique. Summaries of conditions for general consumption may not include all the variations that can be found in individuals. The material you are reading is meant to give you information that can form the basis of your questions, not the final answers. Particularly in rare conditions, there really is a lot that medicine does not know.

Reading long lists of what a condition consists of can sometimes be overwhelming. Not every person may be affected the same way. Make sure to ask questions if something you have read does not seem to apply to your child.

No one is going to know your child as well as you. Make sure to speak up for him or her. The health care professionals may have more experience with the condition, but *you* have more experience with your child.

Love Your Special Child

As is repeated in all parenting books, the role of the parent is to give his or her child unconditional love.[4] Doing so can be harder when you are not getting the usual feedback from your child that parents expect. Part of developing this love is to focus on your child's strengths. Over time many parents learn to get parental joy and satisfaction from smaller steps in their child's development. An often quoted essay that helps put this in perspective is "Welcome to Holland," by Emily Perl Kingsley.[5]

If you were hoping to breastfeed, go ahead. Professional lactation consultants can assist you in breastfeeding a child with special needs. The health benefits of breastfeeding are particularly important for a child who may be hospitalized a number of times and thus will be exposed to hospital-based infections. If the baby is unable to be fed by mouth, breast milk can be expressed and given to the baby via tube feedings. In most metabolic diseases (the sole exception is galactossemia), human milk can be at least part of the diet.

It is scary to love a child who may have a short life span. It is natural to feel that the greater the attachment, the greater the loss. Most parents who have unfortunately lost a child tend be comforted by the memories that they have. Try to make the most of the time that you do have.

Try to "normalize" the situation as much as possible. If your family's custom is to celebrate birthdays, celebrate the birthday of your child with special needs as well. Mark special occasions such as bar/bat mitzvah in a skill-appropriate manner.

As your child gets older, like all other adolescents, he or she may want to have more independence. The website http://www.independentliving. org is a good place to get started in learning how to maneuver the hurdles of independent living with a disability. The website http://www.family village.wisc.edu includes links to other disability websites.

Adults with disabilities have married, had children, held jobs, etc. Depending on your child's condition, help him or her strive for the maximum.

While it is prudent to sit down with professional financial advisors to ensure financial stability for your child when he or she is older,[6] in dealing with your child, don't worry too much about the future—concentrate on enjoying the here and now.

Help Your Special Child

Build a team of specialists to help your child. Depending on your child's needs, you may need some or all of these specialties. Audiologists test hearing. Speech and language pathologists (sometimes called *speech therapists* for short) help in improving speech and communication. Physical therapists help with gross motor skills such as sitting and walking. Occupational therapists tend to focus on fine motor skills, such as writing and manipulation of small objects, as well as on activities of daily living.[7] Feeding issues are generally addressed by either occupational or speech therapists. The goal of all these specialists is to maximize function.

These specialists may be available to you in a number of different settings. Some work individually and some work together as part of a child development clinic. Some of the services may be available to you through your school system. Because the expenditures for various therapies can be substantial over the years, it is important to explore what subsidized care you are eligible for and use personal funds to fill in the gaps for what is not covered.

You play an important role in balancing all the needs of your child—physical, educational, and emotional. It is important to make a list of priorities. Discuss with the professionals what therapies are time sensitive and what, if needed, can wait to a future date. Periodic reevaluation is needed to see what therapy the child can benefit most from.

Children with disabilities may have special health care needs. For example, you want to find a dentist who is comfortable working with your child.[8] These children also have routine health needs such as immunizations. Therefore, it is important to find the physician who can be the case manager for what may be multiple health care issues. This concept is known as the "medical home." At times this person may be the general pediatrician; at other times it may the specialist who knows the condition best.

Educate Your Special Child

Be involved in your child's educational setting. The more the staff of your child's school sees your presence and recognizes your educational input, the more they take the work with your child seriously. Remember to advocate for your child in a positive way. Ask with a smile. Most people who work with children with special needs genuinely want to help.

Families for whom Jewish education is important face additional challenges. On the one hand, public education often provides many services not available in Jewish educational institutions. It also is far less costly, and in smaller Jewish communities it is often the only option. On the other hand, it will not provide a religious education and exposes children to other religious traditions and to a secular lifestyle.

Each family needs to find the proper balance for their child. However, make sure to at least explore local non-Jewish or nonreligious options. At times, formal education in such a setting with supplementation of private lessons in Jewish topics may be the proper option for your child. For other children, formal education in a Jewish school with supplementation of private therapies may be the proper option. Do not hesitate to explore Jewish options that may have a different religious outlook than that of your family. If the school can offer the services your child needs, you can work with him or her to explain why you might do some things a bit differently at home.

Within the Jewish educational system there are a number of choices, depending on your child's level of function or particular disability. These include separate special needs schools,[9] special classes within regular schools, and "mainstreaming"—learning in the regular classroom with additional help as needed.[10] You may need to advocate for your child if you feel he or she could be mainstreamed into the local Jewish school but the school is hesitant. Consultation with organizations such as Kulanu (see previous note) can help the school learn more about this option and how to accommodate your requests.

Help Others Accept Your Child

Make an effort to keep your child well groomed and dressed nicely. While people should be judged on their internal qualities, it is human nature that external appearances matter. Because there is unfortunately a natural tendency to shy away from people who look different, helping your child look more like his or her peers tends to help.

One of the hardest challenges for children with disabilities is finding a social network. You can help by getting it started. Make play dates for your young child just as you would for other children. Don't wait for others to call you. Once they have been at your house, they are likely to reciprocate. Start with short play dates, even 20 minutes at a time. This strategy increases the chances that they will be successful and therefore that they will be repeated.

Planning activities that your child can participate in is a good way to get friendships started. Not every trial is going to work. Even children without disabilities have ups and downs in making friends. However, if you keep on trying, you are doing your best.

As your child gets older, try to get him or her involved in the activities of his or her peer group. This is something that will probably take a fair amount of creativity on your part. For example, if your child is not capable of participating in a competitive sport, perhaps he or she can be the scorekeeper. Speak to leaders of the local teams and shul groups to try to find activities in which your child can participate. It may take a bit of convincing at first, but it is generally worth the effort.

Once your child is going to an activity, don't hover to see how it goes. The child needs room in which to learn and even make mistakes. Yes, there are times when it may be painful. However, these are skills that need to be learned by all children.

There are a number of organizations that plan social activities for children with disabilities. Jewish examples of such organizations are Yachad[11] for the developmentally delayed and Our Way for the deaf. Yachad has camping programs as well, some of which are located within camps for nondisabled children and thus provide a protected place for interaction. The Friendship Circle, run in conjunction with Chabad, helps work specifically on children's social skills.[12]

Being with others similar to oneself, and realizing that one is not alone in dealing with a medical condition, can be very helpful. However, working on interactions in some activities with those without disabilities is also good for children to learn skills.

As your children get older, they may want to have internet contact with others with their condition. This may be particularly helpful for those with rare conditions. In addition to disease-specific chat groups found throughout this book (where applicable), there is a general social hub (http://www.rareshare.org). Of course all safety guidelines for internet usage[13] apply here as well.

When your child gets even older, you may wonder about how to help him or her find a mate—this is a worry of all parents but it is clearly more challenging for those with disabilities. Organizations that assist in social introductions and/or *shidduchim* for individuals with special needs include the Jewish Deaf Singles Registry,[14] Jewish Singles with Special Needs,[15] Singles with Medical Issues Shidduch Group,[16] and Boneh Bayis Shidduchim.[17] However, don't rule out the usual network of friends and family. There are special individuals without disabilities who see beyond disabilities, and there certainly have been marriages in which only one member of the couple has a disability.

Love All Your Children

Find what is special in *all* your children and build on these strengths. Let each one pursue his or her own interests and hobbies and develop individual identities that are separate from "the special child" and "the normal child."

Pay attention to the needs of each child. Even if they don't have a disability, they have needs as well. These include your hearing about their interactions with their friends, their teachers, and siblings, even if their troubles seem minor in comparison to the challenges of your affected child. Let them feel safe saying negative things about their affected sibling without feeling guilty. It may be hard for you to hear it, but it is much better to let them express these negative feelings in words than in actions against either the sibling or themselves or in behavioral difficulties. When there are many children in a large family, this task can be more challenging. However, the presence of a number of siblings without disabilities increases the typical sibling interactions of the unaffected children among themselves.

Spread Your Energies

Care of children requires tremendous time, energy, and patience. The care of a special child needs all this and more. On the other hand, the special child is not the only member of the family who needs attention. Other children, your spouse, and yes, even you, need time and attention as well. Putting on this juggling act is no easy feat.

Actually schedule in time, whether on your iPad or on a notepad. Make sure there is special time that you spend with other family members where they have your full attention. This includes your spouse as well as your other children!

Take Care of Yourself

Even the best-organized parents dealing with a special child are at risk of experiencing burnout. Burnout will make it very hard for you to continue to function at the level needed for the ongoing juggling. Therefore, it is very important to build in time to take care of yourself. If you take care of yourself and portray a positive image, others will mirror your positive attitude and not view you with pity. They will see you for the entire person you are and not just the challenge with which you are dealing.

Building a network of babysitters can help give you time for yourself. Do not consider this a luxury but rather a necessity to allow you to continue in your important task. Some parents are afraid to leave a special needs child in the care of others. However, both extended family and responsible adolescents can be taught the skills they need to babysit for such children. Two useful links for guidance can be found at http://www.suite101.com/article.cfm/babysitting/83570 and http://www.wcdd.org/babysit.html. Students studying therapies or special education often make good babysitters for children with special needs.

The concept of giving families who care for individuals with special needs "a break" is known as *respite care*. There are many organizations that help families with the resources to get this important type of care. A list can be found at http://chtop.org/ARCH/National-Respite-Locator.html. Jewish Family Services (use Google to find your local chapter) or www.jfsisrael.org for Israel can help you find services appropriate for the Jewish community. Camps such as Hebrew Academy for Special Children (HASC) provide this kind of respite care during the summer. In Israel, the Shalva organization runs a number of programs that include family respite.[18]

If you feel that you or a member of your family is becoming overwhelmed, do not hesitate to seek professional counseling. Asking for help is not a sign of weakness; it is a sign of wisdom. The coping techniques that you, your spouse, and/or your children will learn are likely to assist you in many of life's challenges, not only in dealing with a disability.

Parent-to-Parent Support

Parents who are dealing with similar circumstances can be an invaluable resource. They can share methods of handling situations that they have encountered in the day-to-day management of their child's conditions that will not be found in any medical textbook. Almost all the support organizations listed in the sections on specific conditions can help arrange contact with other parents. Your pediatrician may be able to match you up with local families dealing with a similar condition. In addition, there are a number of organizations that can be contacted that deal with a spectrum of rare diseases and resulting disabilities:

Madisons Foundation
PO Box 241956
Los Angeles, CA 90024
Phone: (310) 264-0826
Fax: (310) 264-4766
Email: getinfo@madisonsfoundation.org
Internet: www.madisonsfoundation.org
UK
Contact a Family
Phone: 0808 808 3555
Email: helpline@cafamily.org.uk
Internet: www.cafamily.org.uk
Parent to Parent USA
This is a national organization that lists statewide networks throughout the United States and helps set up parent-to-parent support networks.
Internet: www.p2pusa.org
Exceptional Parent
This is a magazine for parents of children (and adults) with disabilities.
Internet: www.eparent.com
A Different Kind of Perfect: Writings by Parents on Raising a Child with Special Needs by Cindy Dowling[19] is a collection of writing by parents that can also be helpful. Remember, no two families' experiences are the same. However, you can learn a lot (both what to do and not to do) from others.
Specifically for Jewish children with developmental issues and their families:
Yachad, The National Jewish Council for Disabilities
11 Broadway, 13th Floor
New York, NY 10004
Phone: (212) 613-8229
Fax: (212) 613-0796
Email: njcd@ou.org

Kulanu—All of Us
124 McGlynn Place
Cedarhurst, NY 11516
Phone: (516) 569-3083
Fax: (516) 374-1185
Beineinu
U.S. Office
Phone: (347) 743-4900
Email: Golda@beineinu.org
Israel Office
Deena Weinberg
Email: deena@beineinu.org
Phone: 0722305368
Internet: http://beineinu.org
Chai Lifeline
www.chailifeline.org
Website provides information for U.S. regional offices and affiliates in
Canada, the United Kingdom, and Israel.

Remember, parenting is never easy. Hopefully, with the help of Hashem and by drawing on inner strength that you might not even be aware of, you will learn to derive joy from this situation as well. In the words of one mother, "We don't ask for difficulties in life. However, once they are already ours, we can find the challenge very enriching and rewarding—teaching us new lessons and giving us a new appreciation of life."

---

1. "Some children are easy to parent. They rarely get ill, breeze through their milestones precisely on schedule, and are photogenic to boot. The technical term for these youngsters is 'other people's children.'" http://www.childrentoday.com/articles/special-needs/siblings-are-special-too-4268/3.
2. 2:6.
3. Climb Building
   176 Nantwich Road
   Crewe, CW2 6BG
   Phone: 0800 652 3181, 0845 241 2172/2173
   Fax: 0845 241 2174
   General Enquiries: info.svcs@climb.org.uk
   Family Services: fam.svcs@climb.org.uk
   Children and Young Peoples Services: cya.svcs@climb.org.uk

Information Research: ir.svcs@climb.org.uk
Fundraising and Events: frg.svcs@climb.org.uk
Membership Services: mem.svcs@climb.org.uk

4. When dealing with behavioral issues, love and approval are not the same thing. You have the right to express your disapproval of a child's behavior. However, the negative message should be directed to the action, not the child. For example, "It makes me angry to see that you did not follow my instructions," not "You make me angry."

5. Available online at http://www.our-kids.org/Archives/Holland.html. A more "black humor" parody is "Welcome to Beirut," available online at http://www.bbbautism.com/beginners_beirut.htm. An honest poem presenting a different perspective is available online at http://jewishmom.com/2011/09/06/lifes-unspoken-bargains-what-its-really-like-raisinga-special-needs-child-by-anonymous/.

6. A nice summary of issues involved can be found at http://www.ataxia.org/pdf/FinancialPlanning.pdf.

7. In young children, there is sometimes overlap between the specialties.

8. Special Care Dentistry Association
401 North Michigan Avenue
Suite 2200
Chicago, IL 60611
Phone: (312) 527-6764
Fax: (312) 673-6663
Email: scda@scdaonline.org

9. Some examples of such schools are:
The Hebrew Academy for Special Children
5902 14th Ave
Brooklyn, NY 11219
Phone: (718) 686-5912
Fax: (718) 853-0197
Internet: http://www.hasc.net
IVDU Schools run by Yachad, the National Jewish Council for Disabilities
11 Broadway, 13th Floor
New York, NY 10004
Phone: (212) 613-8229
Fax: (212) 613-0796
Email: njcd@ou.org

See section on deafness for Jewish Schools for the Deaf. See Usher Syndrome for Jewish Schools for the Blind.

10. Organizations that assist in arranging the latter two options include:
Kulanu—All of Us
124 McGlynn Place
Cedarhurst, NY 11516

Phone: (516) 569-3083

Fax: (516) 374-1185

Internet: http://www.kulanukids.org/contact.html

The National Association of Day Schools Serving Exceptional Children (NADSEC), hosted by Yachad, the National Jewish Council for Disabilities (contact information above).

11. Both available via the Yachad contact information given at the end of the chapter.

12. The Friendship Circle

6892 West Maple Road

West Bloomfield, MI 48322

Phone: (248) 788-7878

Fax: (248) 788-7854

Internet: www.friendshipcircle.org

13. Such as not giving out personal information and not arranging to meet. In certain situations, meeting may be a possibility, but this should be done only if the contact is made by the parents and supervised at first.

14. http://www.njcd.org/ourway/sections.php?id=C0_70_9.

15. http://www.jswsn.com.

16. FindingOnlyOne@yahoo.com.

17. Phone: (718) 438-1639

18. 6 Ibn Denan Street, PO Box 34449

Jerusalem 91344 Israel

Phone: 02-651-9555

Fax: 02-653-5787

Email: info@shalva.org

19. Random House, 2006.

Welcoming the Disabled Among Us

An important dictum in *Pirkei Avot*[1] is *havei mekabel et kol ha'adam besever panim yafot*, in other words, relate to every person in a pleasant manner. Shammai, the sage quoted here, makes no distinction regarding the level of function of the person being greeted. A recurrent theme stated by parents of children with special needs is the difficulty they have with the reactions of others. A number of mothers have told me that they find it harder to deal with these reactions than with their child's condition. This section is based on the insights and experiences of such parents.

Helping Children with Special Needs
1. Try to treat the children as normally as possible. In many conditions, the child has normal intelligence, even if he or she has an abnormal physical appearance. This is certainly true for such conditions as familial dysautonomia, Bloom syndrome, and Fanconi anemia. Speak to the children the way you would to anyone their age.
2. Try to include them in as many activities with their peers as they are physically capable of. If you are not sure if they are up to it, ask the parents. Even if the child cannot participate in everything being done, just the feeling of being included can go a long way. Genetic diseases are not contagious.
3. Teach your typically developing children how to accept children with special needs. Statements such as "Some of us are born short or tall, some with blue eyes or brown eyes," can help normalize the differences for the young child. Older children can understand the concept that all of us have trouble with *something*.
4. Work with your school, shul, camp, or youth group to see how children with special needs can be included in local activities. One model is to have "shadows"—helpers who can make sure children with special needs can participate in activities such as Shabbat groups. Organizations that assist in arranging this service include Yachad and Kulanu (see section on raising special children for contact information).

Helping Parents of Children with Special Needs

1. Try to treat the parents as normally as possible. Invite them to activities and events just as you would if they did not have a child with special needs.

2. Treat the parents as you would any other friend. It is fine to ask them about their children, including the child with the disability. If you are not yourself familiar with chronic illness or special education, it might take you some time to understand their answers. However, the fact that you are willing to listen helps minimize the isolation that families with special children often experience.

3. Think twice before giving advice. If you have concrete information that you feel would be helpful and appreciated, offer it. If you are asked for your opinion, do give it. Unsolicited advice, however, can be taxing.

4. Care of special children can be very expensive. Think about local *tzedakah* efforts that can be used to help. Remember the principle of *aniyei ircha kodmin*—the poor of your city take precedence.[2] Make sure to determine from the parents (directly or through someone who knows them) the degree of privacy that they wish to maintain.

Helping Make Jewish Institutions Available to Those with Disabilities[3, 4]

The importance of accessibility for those with disabilities has achieved greater public awareness, but there are still many barriers. In 1990 the U.S. Congress passed the Americans with Disabilities Act, which mandates that government facilities and public transportation be accessible to the disabled. In 1998 Israel began to enact similar legislation. Unfortunately, houses of worship are exempt from these laws; a quick look will show how most are not in fact accessible. Things to consider are:

1. Wheelchair access to the shul, the areas of worship (for men and women), and important areas such as the *bimah* and the *aron kodesh*. Wheelchair access to spaces like the bathrooms, *beit midrash*, and social hall is also important. A Shabbat elevator is something to consider when a new shul is designed or an old one renovated.

2. Wheelchair access to the *mikveh*. Lifts to help women unable to walk to use the *mikveh*.

3. Braille and large-print *siddurim* and *chumashim* (available through
    the Jewish Braille Institute).[5] A computer program that translates
    Hebrew texts into Braille via a computer is available for weekday
    use.[6]
4. Sign language interpreters for davening and *shiurim*. Sign lan-
    guage prayer charts.[7]

With effort on all our parts, we can show Hashem that we are truly *am
echad*.

---

1. 1:15.
2. *Bava Metzia* 71a:

ענייך ועניי עירך - ענייך קודמין, עניי עירך ועניי עיר אחרת - עניי עירך קודמין.

This principle also justifies the family's concentrating their own tzedakah efforts
on their child.
3. See also B. S. Brenner, Welcoming Jews with disabilities into Jewish commu-
nal life. *Jewish Action*, Fall 2005: 52–60. Available online at http://www.ou.org/
pdf/ja/5766/fall66/WelcomingJewsDisab.pdf.
4. Full text available online at http://www.ada.gov/pubs/ada.htm.
5. Available through:
     JBI International
     110 East 30th Street
     New York, NY 10016
     Phone: (800) 433-1531
     Fax: (212) 689-3692
     In Israel:
     Mesila Library for the Blind
     Rechov Kehaneman 69
     Bnei Brak
6. Computer Sciences for the Blind (CSB)
     Phone: (718) 837-4549
     http://www.computersciences.org/
7. These can be ordered via:
     Our Way for the Deaf and Hard of Hearing
     The National Jewish Council for Disabilities
     11 Broadway, 13th Floor
     New York, NY 10004
     Phone: (212) 613-8229
     Fax: (212) 613-0796
     Email: njcd@ou.org

Our Way has other resources as well, including a handbook for classroom teachers on the hearing-impaired child in the Jewish classroom.

Effects on the Family
of a Child with Special Needs

Isack Kandel, MA, PhD[a] and Joav Merrick, MD, MMedSci, DMSc[b, 1]

Introduction

When a child joins a family, the life of the family changes significantly; each of its members has to adapt to a new situation. When this child is discovered to have a disability, in addition to the regular adaptive process, the family must cope with many challenges. Sometimes the disability appears at birth in an unexpected manner. At other times, particularly in the cases of genetic diseases that have been diagnosed prenatally, the potential disability is expected before the birth. Sometimes the disability is not suspected until a later age. Regardless of the timing, the news that a child may have a disability often comes as a shock. Different families deal with shock in different ways. For some, it can be experienced as a crisis. Others may reveal significant strengths that allow for good functioning, and yet others can grow from the experience.

The care of the child with a disability requires tapping into many resources. Parents must coordinate assessments, evaluations, and various treatments, maintaining contact with many professionals and numerous institutions or services. They find themselves faced with important decisions on behalf of the child—decisions on management of this new situation, and economic decisions that will affect the whole family. This section is an overview of possible effects on the family unit of the birth of a child with special health needs.

Impact on the Parents as Individuals

The realization that a child has a disability can cause a number of reactions in the parents. These will vary from couple to couple; even the two parents of the same child will not respond identically. The intensity of reactions and their character depend on several dynamic factors, such as personality, the character of social relations, feelings about the condition, and social status. Furthermore, the coping process is not static but rather a constantly changing cognitive and behavioral effort by the person to manage both external and internal stress factors and pressures.

Realizing that it is common to have negative reactions can help parents search for help in dealing with them. Some parents will find that the support of friends or the community is sufficient. Others will find elements of religion such as prayer to be helpful in rising above these feelings. The many support organizations listed throughout this book can help reach out to other parents who have gone through similar experiences. Should these alone not be sufficient, parents should not hesitate to seek professional psychological support.

The following are common reactions. Not everyone will experience them. However, if you do experience them, know that you are not alone.

Disappointment
Disappointment that the child will not fulfill the parents' expectations is a common initial reaction.[2] Many parents have questions such as *why did this happen to me* or *what did I do wrong to deserve this*? For religious couples, this feeling may lead to questions of faith.

Psychological Stress
Some parents may feel significant psychological stress from the diagnosis. This may result in low self-esteem, shame, embarrassment, anger, or jealousy.

There may be unconscious manifestations of this stress, resulting in anger directed toward oneself, or toward those professionals caring for the child. The emotions may also be directed toward other families, who do not have to contend with such stress, or toward those with disabled children who are higher functioning or have improved to a greater extent. Sometimes the opposite reaction can be observed, which is expressed in overprotecting the child.

Grief
Because realizing that a child has a disability involves the loss of the "ideal" child that parents had imagined, the initial diagnosis of the child's disability will often produce a grief reaction in parents and other family members.[3] Many families seem to go through the five stages of Kubler-Ross grief elaboration theory (denial, anger, bargaining, depression, and acceptance).[4, 5, 6] It is important to realize that these stages are variable; different people will experience them in different order, and not all parents

will experience all of them. These stages are also dynamic; a person can go back and forth between stages. It is also important to realize that there can be gender differences in the parental response to the situation.[7]

As the child grows older, birthdays or other rites of passage (e.g., siblings celebrating bar/bat mitzvahs, being drafted into the army, graduating, or getting married) may underscore how different the child is from his typical peers. On the other hand, many parents learn over time how to derive joy from minor advances that would not be noticed at all in a child without a disability.

Emotions tend to be to be most intense with the sudden change of reality at the time of diagnosis. Later, many parents find themselves dealing with ambivalent feelings. They vacillate between parental feelings of love for their child and worry about societal reactions to their child.

Parents also need to deal with the objective difficult conditions of bringing up a child with special health needs. Focusing on practical approaches to the issue can help return a sense of control. Learning as much as possible about the suspected or known diagnosis of the child also helps many families cope. Support organizations can be helpful in providing information about the condition and guidance for accessing any governmental or organizational assistance available to help in dealing with the new reality. Over time, many families are able to redefine their expectations and rebuild around the new reality.

Frustration

Frustration with the situation is a common reaction. It can become even deeper as the slow development of the child leads to a wider and wider gap between the child and his or her peers. If the child is dependent on his parents for activities of daily living, this responsibility can markedly affect the parents' independence and freedom, especially the mother's. Disabilities in a child can cause difficulties in maintaining social communication, leisure activities, work projects, or economic plans.

The degree of frustration can be lessened with planning. In order to make the best of a challenging situation, it is important that the parents openly discuss their roles. While the main caregiving role will tend to fall on one parent, efforts should be made by the other parent to assume at least some aspects of the care. To prevent burnout, it is quite important that respite time be built into the family schedule for the primary caretaker. Resources of the extended family and community can make a major impact on the functioning of the nuclear family. While it is hard for many parents to overcome the difficulty of asking others for help, or sharing the fact that they are stressed, the long-term rewards of having such assistance merit dealing with the initial embarrassment.

Guilt

Guilty feelings are among the most frequent reactions of the parents to the birth of a child with a disability. This feeling has sometimes been caused by the medical and professional community, who directly or inadvertently attributed a disease or condition in a child as parental failure though it later turned out to be based on a genetic disorder. Many parents wonder if they unwittingly did something to contribute to the disability in their child (such as exposure to X-rays, mercury from injections, or dental fillings). Recognizing that this reaction of guilt is common is the first step in preventing negative consequences of such feelings.

In summary, strong reactions by parents, many of them difficult, are likely upon hearing of the possibility of a disability in a child. However, there are families who voluntarily adopt children with disabilities, showing the variability of family coping mechanisms.

Recognizing that these reactions are common and getting help in dealing with them is the best way to ensure that one's family adjusts to the new reality in the best possible manner. Parents can turn to each other, their extended family, and other positive resources (friend, rabbi, or counselor) to communicate their feelings and frustrations and to get practical help, information, and advice and understand that they are not alone.

Impact on the Parents as a Couple

Having a child with special needs can put stress on a marriage. [8, 9, 10]

One frequent problem is the fact that burden of child care is not divided equally between the parents. The father is generally at work while the mother cares for the child with the disability. To help prevent the burning out of one partner, parents should organize a system of roles and a division of the burden of work.[11] Time should be put aside for the couple to spend together unrelated to the needs of the child (or other children). Sometimes the conflict stems from the fact that each parent perceives the situation in a different way. One parent may relate to the child as a failed case while the other sees him as a capable, or even a normal, child. Professional counseling can help the couple find legitimate expression for their feelings and reduce the extent to which these feelings become a source of conflict.

It is important to realize that each person will adjust in different ways and at a different pace. To help learn to cope together:

- Talk openly about problems and issues that need to be solved.
- Use friends and family to provide extra support and build a family support network.
- Spend time together alone for rest and recreation.
- Be patient.
- Take care of yourself.
- Celebrate events in the life of the child.
- Participate in family events with the child as part of the family.

It is important for couples to facilitate good communication, learn to listen, maintain respect and trust, keep a sense of humor, and know when they need help from others (family, friends, and/or professionals).

The most important point is to not give up. Take life one day at a time and continue to have a positive outlook on life. Traditional Jewish sources[12] encourage us to believe that there is a reason for everything, even though we do not always understand what it is.

Impact on Grandparents and Other Members of the Extended Family

In some families grandparents are a major resource and support. This can be especially true with a grandchild with a disability. In our modern society we are not always fortunate enough to have grandparents close by, and distance will prevent them from taking an active role in daily life. But wherever they are, it is important that they support and encourage the parents, brothers, and sisters, and they can serve as role models, sources of information, and trusted confidants.

Grandparents can serve as "time out" for parents, sibling(s), and the child with the disability, but this feasibility depends on the disability, and on the ability of the grandparents to cope. Grandparents certainly also have important roles in family events (holidays, bar/bat mitzvah, weddings, etc.), when they can be a support and help.

On the other hand, sometimes well-meaning family can be "too much." It is important to have open communication with members of the family to lay out guidelines as to what the parents perceive as help and what they perceive as meddling.

Impact on Siblings

A number of studies have shown that having a disabled sibling has an impact on the other children in the family.[13, 14, 15] The degree of impact can vary according to the disability.[16]

The concerns of the children may be varied. In one study of siblings of children with physical disabilities (43 children), the siblings reported difficulties with common activities and communication with the disabled sibling as well as concern for the future and the health of their disabled sibling.[17] In this study, having a sibling with a disability did not affect relationships with friends. A study that looked at the attitude of the child toward the brother or sister found that some of the very young children wanted to be similar and tried to imitate their disabled sibling, especially if the sibling had a physical disability.[18] Even before the age of two years, children were able to recognize that their brother or sister was different and often imitated the parents' behavior toward the older child.

A four-year follow-up study among Orthodox Jewish families (82 families) in Illinois showed an increase in sibling and overall family adjustment over time. Parents cited religion as an important source of strength.[19] Some parents felt that the siblings of disabled children developed increased sensitivity to people with special needs and a greater appreciation for the "normal" things in life.

In the past, families sometimes kept the existence of a child with a disability a secret, even to the point where children did not know they had a sibling in residential care. This approach is generally not helpful. When the siblings know about the existence of the disabled child, either at home or in out-of-home care, some will become quite protective. If the siblings want to be involved in the care, they should be allowed do so in an age-appropriate manner. On the other hand, children need their own space and should not be forced to take on the role of caregiver.

To help your other children, it is important to be aware of the effects that a disabled child can have on a sibling and to:
- make sure you give room to the sibling(s) to express their feelings to you, and take the time needed to listen to them.
- make quality time to be with the sibling(s).
- make sure the sibling(s) have their own activities and leisure time.
- encourage the sibling(s) to invite friends over to visit.

Impact on the Child with the Disability

As he or she gets older, the child with a disability will have to cope with the challenges faced in growing up. Some of these are faced by all children his age. Others will be unique and due to the disability. The child will need to learn adaptive coping mechanisms. Parents can best help their children by learning all they can about the disability as soon as they can. They should treat the child as a regular member of the family, including helping out with chores to the best of his or her ability. With realistic expectations of what can be achieved, they should work to give their child every opportunity to grow. Contacting the many support groups and professional organizations can help them learn from others how to do this.

Child Rearing

Why reinvent the wheel? It is recommended that parents with a disabled child seek out other parents who have been through the same life events and get support, help, and advice. The internet is a rich resource for access to such parents. In addition to the many resources mentioned throughout this book, search for "special children," "special needs kids," "parenting," or combinations. Many common concerns are addressed in this book in the section on A Special Kind of Parenthood.

Education

Special needs education means the special educational arrangements that are in place for people with disabilities. All children, including those with disabilities and those with special needs, have a right to free primary education. Children with special educational needs have the right to free primary education up to age 18–21 years, depending on the country. Most countries today try to provide special needs education in mainstream settings as far as possible. Education for children with special needs may be provided in ordinary classes in mainstream schools, in special classes in mainstream schools, or in special schools or home schooling.

As parents you should make sure that your child is assessed for special educational needs and has a personal education plan. Depending on the country where you live, there are usually special transport arrangements, including escorts and safety measures, available for disabled children attending school.

Transition to Adulthood

As a result of advances in treatment over the last three decades (e.g., pharmacology, surgical techniques, medical technology), the life expectancy for young adults with many types of serious conditions that were once fatal in childhood is 30, 40, and sometimes 60 years.

On the other hand, the advances in medical science have not been matched by advances in the organization, financing, and delivery of care for these young adults. In the late 1980s, experts in the provision of health care to children with chronic health and developmental needs recognized that pediatric providers and facilities could not adequately address the medical and related needs of the rapidly growing and ever-aging population of young people with special health care needs. In response to this emerging problem, the U.S. Surgeon General convened the "Growing up and getting medical care: Youth with special health care needs" conference in 1989. This group proposed the following key actions:

- Recognize the importance of starting the transition process early.
- Promote the autonomy and self-management skills of adolescents.
- Educate pediatricians about promising transition practices.
- Build bridges between pediatric and adult medicine.
- Provide adult-oriented physicians with training in the management of childhood-onset conditions.

In the years that followed, numerous professional and provider organizations and advocacy groups developed consensus statements and planning documents that affirm and build on these core goals and activities. However, a multiplicity of problems, issues, and barriers has impeded efforts to implement these plans and make successful transition systems a reality. Other countries also tend to lag in providing for smooth transition to adult care for children with disabilities.

It is therefore very important for every family with a disabled child to inquire about relevant adult services before the child reaches 18–21 years of age, in order to ensure a smooth transition to an optimal and continuous health care provision.

Out-of-Home Placement

Care for a disabled child at home has become a more common option than residential care.[20] For example, an in-depth study of 167 Australian families of young children with a disability with a qualitative in-depth investigation of the everyday family life experiences showed that 75 percent definitely did not want to place their child, 19 percent were undecided, and 6 percent were actively seeking or had already sought placement. The factors that influenced placement were the conflict between the needs of the child and those of other family members, lack of integration of the child in everyday family life and the community, and a concern about the effect of the child on the siblings now and in the future.[21]

Many parents who at first chose home care find it harder to have their disabled child at home when they and the child grow older,[22] especially when further health problems occur.[23] If the social welfare system provides suitable care for aging persons with intellectual disability living at home, the affected person will stay longer at home or even in independent living. Sometimes a decline in the health and functioning of the child will force the parents to seek out-of-home placement.

Families with high levels of financial resources were more likely to plan for the child to continue living at home.[24] Out-of-home placement is an ongoing process, and once the idea of placement is entertained, it still takes several years to act upon.[25]

Conclusions

This chapter looked at the effects on the family unit of the realization that a child has a disability. This event can have major impact on the family. However, with early and sensitive care and intervention for the involved child, the parents, and siblings, much can be done to help the family. This support can help the family to adjust and become positively involved in the care and development of the child, even if that child is in need of special care.[26]

1. [a]National Institute of Child Health and Human Development, Office of the Medical Director, Division for Mental Retardation, Ministry of Social Affairs, Jerusalem, Israel, and [b]Kentucky Children's Hospital, University of Kentucky, Lexington. Correspondence: Professor Joav Merrick, MD, MMedSci, DMSc, Medical Director, Division for Mental Retardation, Ministry of Social Affairs, PO Box 1260, IL-91012 Jerusalem, Israel. Email: jmerrick@zahav.net.il

2. W. Wolfensberger and R. A. Kurtz, eds. *Management of the Family of the Mentally Retarded.* River Grove, IL: Follett Educational Corp., 1969.

3. A. Ross. *The Exceptional Child in the Family.* New York: Grune and Stratton, 1964.

4. E. Kubler-Ross. *On Death and Dying.* New York: Macmillan, 1969.

5. C. Calandra, G. Finocchiaro, L. Raciti, and A. Alberti. Grief elaboration in

families with handicapped member. *Ann. Ist. Super Sanita* 1992: 28, 269–71.

6. R. J. Harmon, N. S. Plummer, and K. A. Frankel, Perinatal loss: Parental grieving, family impact and intervention services. In: J. D. Osofsky and H. E. Fitzgerald, eds. *Handbook of Infant Mental Health.* New York: John Wiley, 2000; 4, 327–68.

7. A. Sullivan, Gender differences in coping strategies of parents of children with Down syndrome. *Down Syndr. Res. Pract.* 2002 8 (2), 67–73.

8. C. M. Fowle, The effect of the severely mentally retarded child on his family. *Am. J. Ment. Defic.* 1968; 73:468–73.

9. B. J. Tew, K. M. Laurence, H. Payne, and K. Rawnsley, Marital stability following the birth of a child with spina bifida. *Br. J. Psychiatry* 1977; 131, 79–82.

10. H. Featherstone. *A Difference in the Family: Life with a Disabled Child.* New York: Basic Books, 1980.

11. P. Withers and L. Bennett, Myths and marital discord in a family with a child with profound physical and intellectual disabilities. *Br. J. Learning Disabil* 2003; 31, 91–95.

12. In the Tanach there is the book of Job. More recent reading on the topic "why is this happening to me" can be found in books such as *Reasonable Doubts: A Religious Skeptic Learns a Thing or Two About God.* Jerusalem: Urim Publications, 2010.

13. N. Breslau, Siblings of disabled children: Birth order and age-spacing effects. *J. Abnorm. Child Psychol.* 1982; 10:85–96.

14. A. Gath and D. Gumley, Retarded children and their siblings. *J. Child Psychol. Psychiatry* 1987; 28:715–30.

15. L. Dyson, E. Edgar, and K. Crnic, Psychological predictors of adjustment by siblings of developmentally disabled children. *Am. J. Ment. Retard.* 1989; 94:292–302.

16. S. Fisman, L. Wolf, D. Ellison, and T. Freeman, A longitudinal study of siblings of children with chronic disabilities. *Can. J. Psychiatry* 2000; 45:369–75.

17. I. M. Pit-Ten Cate and G. M. Loots, Experiences of siblings of children with physical disabilities: an empirical investigation. *Disabil. Rehabil.* 2000; 22:399–408.

18. A. Hames, Do younger siblings of learning-disabled children see them as similar or different? *Child Care Health Dev.* 1998; 24:157–68.

19. Y. Leyser, Stress and adaptation in Orthodox Jewish families with a disabled child. *Am. J. Orthopsychiatry* 1994; 64:376-85.

20. An interesting study performed in Aberdeen, United Kingdom (D. May and J. Hogg, Continuity and change in the use of residential services by adults with intellectual disability: the Aberdeen cohort at mid-life. *J. Intelect. Disabil. Res.* 2000; 44:68–80) reported on a follow-up of a representative cohort of people with intellectual disability born between the years 1951 and 1955. At the age of 22, 60 percent (44 persons) were living at home with their parents and 40 percent

were in residential care (29 persons). At age 40, the most significant change was the increase in the percentage of those cared for at home, which accounted for half of the surviving cohort (24 out of 54 persons), 20 still living at home and 10 in hospital/long-term care. Out-of-home placements were associated with gender (male), challenging behavior, and the absence of one or both parents.

21. G. Llewellyn, P. Dunn, M. Fante, L. Turnbull, and R. Grace, Family factors influencing out-of-home placement decisions. *J. Intellect. Disabil. Res.* 1999; 43:219–33.

22. A. Rimmerman, Out of home placement among families of children with developmental disability. Research perspective (Hebrew). *Society Welfare* 1994; 14:329–42.

23. H. Lifshitz and J. Merrick, Ageing and intellectual disability in Israel: a study to compare community residence with living at home. *Health Soc. Care Community* 2003; 11:364–71.

24. D. A. Cole and L. H. Meyer, Impact of needs and resources on family plans to seek out-of-home placement. *Am. J. Ment. Retard.* 1989; 93:380–87.

25. J. Blacher, Assessing placement tendency in families with children who have severe handicaps. *Res. Dev. Disabil.* 1990; 11:349–59.

26. Recommended further reading: J. Singer. *The Special Needs Parent Handbook: Critical Life Strategies to Help you Survive and Thrive*. New Jersey, self-published 2009.

Halachic Living with Genetic Conditions

For the *halacha*-observant person and family, management of the symptoms of genetic conditions needs to be incorporated into a halachic lifestyle. The goal of this section is to give an overview of halachic aspects of symptoms, treatments, and adaptive devices associated with various diseases and disabilities. Since the range of disabilities and symptoms is broad, and the degree to which individuals are affected varies, this section should be approached as an overview, not a comprehensive compendium.[1]

It should be remembered that *halacha* is case specific. Therefore, for practical guidance an individual question should be asked of a halachic authority.[2] It is very important, however, to ask the question appropriately. A proper answer needs to be based on proper information. Therefore, the halachic authority should be given the most up-to-date information about the person's condition and the medical impact of the situation being asked about. The medical professionals also need to understand the importance of Jewish law in the life of the affected person. Ideally, the medical and halachic professionals will talk to each other directly. If not, the family may have to act as the go-between. Written letters that convey the important information can be helpful in facilitating inter-professional communication.

One of the challenges in trying to find out what to do in specific situations is the lack of modern published material. Reading through traditional sources can give one an incorrect view of proper practice. Two such examples can be found in the cases of blindness and deafness.

In the Talmud (*Kiddushin* 31a) a story is related regarding Rav Yosef Bar Chiya, who lived in the mid third century CE in Babylonia, where, although blind, he served as the head of the Pumbeditha Yeshiva. He states:

> At first I thought: If someone tells me that the *halacha* follows the opinion of Rabbi Yehuda, who said: A blind person is exempt from the commandments, I will make a party—because I am not obligated and I observe the commandments [and thus must be deserving of "extra credit"]. Now that I have heard the statement of Rabbi Chanina that one who is obligated in

commandments and keeps them is greater than one who is not obligated in commandments and keeps them—on the contrary! Whoever tells me that the *halacha* does *not* follow the opinion of Rabbi Yehuda, I will make a party.

Reading this story, which is often taught as part of a discussion of women's exemption from time-bound commandments, would lead one to believe that the blind are exempt. However, the final *halacha* is that the blind are obligated in all commandments other than those in which seeing is an integral part of the commandment. Despite statements that a blind person could not be a member of the Sanhedrin, he can be a member of a rabbinic court (*beit din*). In the past, when the man who was called up to the Torah read the verses that comprised his *aliyah*, a blind person could not perform this role. Today, however, when there is generally a designated reader (*baal korei*) for everyone, a blind man can be given an *aliyah*.[3]

Another example that has undergone transformation is deafness. The Mishna generally lists the *cheresh*, the deaf person, together with the *katan* (minor) and the *shoteh* (insane person)[4] as three categories of people who lack the necessary understanding for the performance of many commandments and halachic obligations. In *Chagiga* 2b however, the Talmud clarifies that this restriction refers only to one who can neither speak nor hear, and therefore cannot communicate with others.[5] With the advent of sign language, it was debated if being able to communicate in this language would count as speaking. The overall consensus today is that it does, and a deaf person who can communicate is fully obligated in the commandments.[6, 7] Furthermore, one who can hear with a hearing aid or cochlear implant can fulfill the commandments for which hearing is needed, similar to the way one who needs glasses or has undergone cataract surgery can fulfill the commandments for which seeing in needed.

Using the term *shoteh* to describe the insane person leaves a gap for a halachic category for the intellectually challenged who are not insane. Some sources have applied the term *shoteh* to mental incapacity in addition to mental illness. The Rambam,[8] however, introduces another term, *peti*, for one who is mentally retarded. He also uses the terminology of *peti beyoter* for one who is severely retarded. Individual rulings are needed to determine a person's mental ability for purposes of obligation in the commandments.

The education of one who is mentally retarded is required according to his ability. If the mental deficiency is very severe, there is no obligation.[9] However, if the child functions well enough cognitively to understand that God gave us the Torah, skill-appropriate education should be given.[10, 11]

Participation in special education programs arranged by Jewish organizations such as Yachad help meet this obligation. It is also possible to work with the child's general education teachers to ensure that what he or she is being taught also has Jewish content. Just as children with special educational needs have individual education programs (IEPs) for their general education, a similar program of skill appropriate mitzvah education and expectation can be worked out with halachic consultation. Periodical reassessment should also be done to account for progress over time. This program should include education toward the true meaning of bar/bat mitzvah, the point at which one becomes obligated to keep the commandments.

When necessary, *halacha* provides much leeway to allow those with disabilities to participate in community activities.[12] In the words of Rabbi Moshe Tendler and Dr. Fred Rosner:

> Jewish law exempts the disabled from any guilt they might feel because of their inability to perform certain commandments, thus affirming that the basic worth and spirituality of the disabled is not diminished in any way. *Halachah* urges them to achieve their fullest potential as Jews while exhorting society to assist them in making their religious observance possible.[13]

Rav Moshe Feinstein, in a responsum where he permits allowing a seeing eye dog into shul, states: "There is no greater need than this because otherwise he will be kept his entire life from public prayer, Torah reading and Megillah reading in public." There is also significant leeway for the disabled on Shabbat.[14] Despite the fact that hearing aids are electronic, they may be worn on Shabbat. While they should not be adjusted over Shabbat, they can be put on and removed, and one should not hesitate to talk to a person wearing one.[15] While there are halachic issues in the use of animals on Shabbat, a blind person can use a seeing eye dog. The same stands to reason for other assistance animals if the person is not mobile without them. There is debate about the permissibility of holding the dog's harness and going out in an area that does not have an *eruv*.[16] A blind person who cannot walk without a stick,[17] or a person who needs a cane or walker, may use them even where there is no *eruv*. Although another Jew cannot push a wheelchair in such an area, a non-Jew can do so.[18] Special adaptations can be made to much adaptive equipment to allow its use on Shabbat to enhance mobility and the Shabbat experience of the disabled or ill.[19]

One of the guiding principles in determining what can be done on Shabbat for a person with health issues emerges from the concepts of *choleh she'yesh bo sakanah* and *choleh she'ein bo sakanah*. The first refers to one who is at medical risk, the second is still ill but not at risk. For someone in the first category, all activities normally prohibited on Shabbat, even on a Torah level, can be performed. However, when it is known that a person is going to need equipment over Shabbat, it is best to arrange to have it run in a way to prevent such activities, such as having it be turned on indirectly with a timer or with special delayed switches. When care is needed for someone who is in the second category, one is allowed to ask a non-Jew to perform any normally prohibited activity. For many of the genetic diseases discussed in this book, there is an underlying medical instability that would qualify the person, even when doing well, as a *choleh she'yesh bo sakanah*. Individual questions should always be asked.

There is an additional category of illness on Shabbat known as *mechash be'alma*, or a minor complaint. In that context, taking medication on Shabbat is not permitted. Most medications for chronic illnesses would not fall into this category, especially when they are taken on a daily basis. However, some nutritional supplements, where skipping a dose might not matter, may be best left to take after Shabbat. Here too, individual questions should be asked.

Physical therapy is also considered a form of healing. In general, physical therapy exercises for the basically healthy should be done before or after Shabbat. One should consult with the therapist as to the impact of not doing such exercises on Shabbat. Where skipping the exercises would have a deleterious effect on a significantly ill person, then it would be permitted. Again, individual questions should be asked.

Many children with severe disabilities are fed by gastrostomy (feeding) tube. Food delivered in this manner does not have to be kosher.[20] It is also not defined as "eating" with regard to Yom Kippur. If one is physically unable to eat normally, one is exempt from commandments related to eating. In cases of severely restricted diets, a specific question should be asked. For those with swallowing issues, wetting and mashing bread or grinding matzah are possible ways to allow fulfillment of relevant commandments. Consultation with an oral function therapist can help people for whom such eating is a problem, and who are troubled by their inability to fulfill the mitzvah.

Bleeding disorders can raise halachic questions. Keeping *hilchot niddah* can be a challenge for women with such disorders. It is important to realize that not all vaginal bleeding makes a woman *niddah* and that specific questions should be asked.[21] If a baby boy is known to have a bleeding disorder, consultation with a hematologist before the *brit milah* can help provide the medical support needed to allow the performance of the procedure.

People with disabilities, like other members of the community, see marriage and family as a central part of their role as adults.[22] For the physically disabled, there is no halachic impediment to marriage. For the intellectually disabled, if the couple is mentally capable of understanding the concept of marriage, then marriage is possible as well. Women with either physical or mental disabilities may need help in the performance of some aspects of *hilchot niddah*.[23]

Consideration as to the ability of the couple to raise children should be part of decisions regarding contraception for the couple. However, this needs to be individualized to the skills of the couple and the outside help that can be provided. It should not be assumed that it is not possible. In cases of genetic disorders, the inheritance of the condition should be part of the decision as well. Up-to-date genetic information should be obtained and conveyed to the halachic authority advising the couple. It should also be remembered that Judaism encourages marriage even in cases where childbearing is not possible.

In summary, it should always be remembered that people affected by genetic diseases are people. For Jewish people affected by genetic diseases, their Judaism may well be an important part of their identity. Therefore, continued work is needed to ensure that their needs are met in this area.

---

1. A practical summary, *Familial Dysautonomia and Jewish Law*, was written by Rabbi Yaakov Eizenbach. While the book discusses halachic issues in the care of those with FD, the topics that it covers (use of adaptive equipment on Shabbat, prayer when one is incapacitated, etc.) are relevant for many other genetic diseases with a neurological component. It can be ordered at http://www.familial-dysautonomia.org/news/Publications.htm.

An academic compendium is: T. C. Marx. *Disability in Jewish Law (Jewish Law in Context)*. London & New York: Routledge, 2002.

2. One such resource is Rav Shaul Anvari, an Orthodox rabbi in Israel who is differently-abled, having been born with cerebral palsy. Questions can be sent to him via http://shaul-anvari.info/contact. Some responses can be found on his blog: http://shaul-anvari.info. He is also currently working on a book of such responsa.

3. For further discussion, see C. Friedman, Haiver behalacha. *Michlol* 2007; 14. Available at www.daat.ac.il.

4. The Talmud in *Chagiga* 3b describes the erratic behavior of the *shoteh*. For this reason, *shoteh* is translated as "insane." For further discussion of the shoteh as a form of mental illness, see R. Strous, Halachic sensitivity to the psychotic individual: the *shoteh*. *Jewish Medical Ethics*. Available online at www.medethics.org.il/articles/JME/JMEB1/JMEB1.21.asp.

5. *Chagiga* 2b states:

> A deaf person who is similar to an insane person or a minor. Just as the minor and the insane person do not have legal mental capacity, so the deaf person does not have legal mental capacity. This is to teach us that the deaf person that the sages spoke about in all places is one who can neither hear nor speak. One who speaks but does not hear, or hears and does not speak, is obligated in the commandments. Thus it is taught: One who speaks and does not hear is a deaf person, one who hears and does not speak is a mute person, and both are considered of normal mental capacity for all purposes.

6. B. Lau, Disability and Judaism: Society's Influence on Halacha. Available at http://jewishdisabilityunite.wordpress.com/2010/01/28/disability-and-judaism-societys-influence-on-halacha-rabbi-dr-benjamin-lau/.

7. See also J. D. Bleich, Status of the Deaf Mute in Jewish Law. *Contemporary Halachic Problems* Vol. 2. New York: Ktav Publishing House, 1983, pp. 368–75.

8. *Rambam Hilchot Edut* 9:10.

9. H. Lifshitz and J. Merrick, Jewish Law and the Definition of Mental Retardation: The Status of People with Intellectual Disability Within the Jewish Law in Relation to the 1992 AAMR Definition of Mental Retardation. *Journal of Religion, Disability and Health* 2001; 5:39–51.

10. J. D. Bleich, Torah Education of the Mentally Retarded. *Contemporary Halachic Problems* Vol. 2. New York: Ktav Publishing House, 1983, 300–310.

11. M. Taubes, Chinuch and the Special Needs Child. Lecture Yeshiva University, February 12, 2008. http://www.yutorah.org/lectures/lecture.cfm/722097/Rabbi_Michael_Taubes/Chinuch_and_the_Special_Needs_Child.

12. M. D. Tender and F. Rosner, The physically and mentally disabled: insights based on the teachings of Rav Moshe Feinstein. *Journal of Halacha and Contemporary Society* 1991; 22. Available online at www.daat.ac.il/daat/english/halacha/tendler_1.htm. Accessed November 9, 2010.

13. *Iggrot Moshe, Orach Chaim* 1:45:

שאין שעה"ד גדול מזה שאם לא נתירנו יתבטל כל ימיו מתפלה בצבור וקה"ת וקריאת המגילה
בצבור וגם יש ימים שהעגמת נפש גדולה מאד כגון בימים נוראים וכה"ג שרבים מתאספים עיין
ברמ"א /או"ח/ ס"ס פ"ח, שלכן ראיה גדולה שיש להתיר להסומא שהכלב שמוליכו צריך להיות
אצלו תמיד, ליכנס לביהכ"נ להתפלל ולשמוע קה"ת וכדומה.

14. See the chapter on Welcoming the Disabled Among Us as to the need for Jewish society to provide more access.

15. For a full discussion of the use of hearing aids on Shabbat, see E. Sandler, The use of hearing aids on Shabbat. *Journal of Halacha and Contemporary Society* 2001; 41. Available online at www.dda.ac.il/daat/english/journal/sandler-1.htm.

16. A. Steinberg, *Encyclopedia Refuit Hilchatit sv. Iver.*

17. Magen Avraham on *Shulchan Aruch Orach Chaim*, 301:18.

18. *Iggrot Moshe, Orach Chaim* 4:90.

19. Switches of this kind, either separately or built into equipment, can be ordered via Machon Tzomet: http://www.zomet.org.il/Eng/?CategoryID=248.

20. *Orach Chaim* 2:88, *Yoreh Deah* 2:59.

21. See www.yoatzot.org.

22. S. Piron, Hama'amad hachuki ve hahilchati shel nesuie zugot im mugbaluyot. Available online at www.ypt.co.il/print.asp?id=30834.

23. D. Zimmerman, The participation of disabled women in the rules of niddah. *Journal of Religion, Disability and Health* 2007; 10:217–20.

Death of a Child

Despite advances in the treatment of many genetic diseases, a number of the conditions described in this book still lead to death in childhood. Therefore, sad as the topic is, this book would not be complete without some discussion of the end of life.

Most of the research on the topic of death in children surrounds sudden death, especially sudden infant death syndrome (SIDS). As is indicated from the name, this experience is somewhat different from that of death from a genetic disease, where the outcome is generally known from the time of diagnosis. The most comparable situation to death from genetic diseases is death from childhood cancer. In cancer, the death is generally anticipated, and there have been major advances in providing hospice care to help families cope with such deaths. However, the issues of end-of-life cancer care—primarily pain control—are not necessarily the same as the neurological decline that typifies many genetic diseases with childhood fatality.[1] For example, an additional consideration in genetic diseases is that there may be another affected child in the household. Facing the death of one child emphasizes the fragility of the other affected child(ren). If the other children are cognizant enough of the death, they are brought face to face with their own fragility as well.[2][3]

Despite the lack of written material, many multidisciplinary teams that deal with potentially fatal conditions have specialists whose role is to help families, and the child involved, deal with impending demise. The expertise of these specialists, known as *thanologists*, can be helpful to many families in dealing with this difficult situation. Most thanologists and others who specialize in hospice care are sensitive to the religious needs of the families they help. Teamwork with the family's rabbi can help deal with specifically Jewish issues that may arise.

Toward the End
Parents of a child with a degenerative genetic disease may well be faced with the kinds of end-of-life decisions generally discussed in the care of adults. These can include which medical interventions to allow and which to refuse. A full discussion of end-of-life decisions is beyond the scope of this book. However, seeing some classic sources used in the

discussion of the topic is important in understanding the parameters on which individual halachic decisions are based.

Judaism places significant emphasis on the value of life, even temporary life. This viewpoint can be seen from the Mishna (*Yoma* 8:7), which states that if someone is trapped under rubble, one may violate all the prohibitions of Shabbat in order to save him, even if one is not sure that he is alive. The *mishna* continues to say that if one finds him alive, one continues, and if he is dead, then one leaves the body until after Shabbat. This instruction to continue seems redundant. The Talmud (*Yoma* 85a) infers from this redundancy that even if it is obvious that he will live for only a few moments, we still continue to do activities normally forbidden on Shabbat as part of the rescue mission, since even a few moments of life are precious. This injunction to transgress Shabbat prohibitions for even temporary life is codified as *halacha* by the *Shulchan Aruch*.[4] As was explained by Rabbi Yisrael Meir HaCohen in his halachic work *Mishna Brura*, even if the person has a clearly fatal injury from the collapse, we still do whatever we can to save him, including activities normally prohibited on Shabbat.[5]

Legally, a dying person (a *goses*) has all the rights of someone who is alive. We are enjoined not to do anything that might hasten the death of such a person. The Mishna[6] lists the actions that may not be performed. As codified by the *Shulchan Aruch*,[7] one is limited in the actions that one can do with a dying person for fear that these actions will hasten the death.

On the other hand, Judaism does not feel there is a need for unchecked, prolonged suffering.[8] The Talmud in *Ketubot* 104a relates the story of the day of the death of Rabbi Yehuda Hanasi. The rabbis were praying to keep him alive and were succeeding. However, his maidservant saw how much he was suffering. She took a vessel and threw it down from the roof to the ground, where it smashed. The noise startled the rabbis into stopping their prayers for a few seconds, and at that point Rabbi Yehuda Hanasi died.

Deciding what is the halachically correct course to take for a terminally ill patient requires balancing the principle of the sanctity of life with the principle of not prolonging suffering. A key point is that this idea refers to the suffering of the patient himself, not necessarily those around him. Not continuing to prolong life is based on reducing suffering, not on judgments as to the quality of life. The Mishna in *Sanhedrin* 4:5, which stresses the need to save even one person, makes no distinction as to the person's level of function. Thus the question of prolonging suffering comes into play when the patient is in severe pain. It is not relevant if the patient is permanently unconscious and unaware of his surroundings but does not seem to be experiencing discomfort. While it may be obvious to those who have grown up on Torah values that this is the case, it is illustrative to see that such an approach was not the standard of society at the time that the Mishna was written.[9]

Active euthanasia of terminally ill children is part of medical discourse in modern society as well. Holland has protocols that allow active euthanasia.[10] A prominent Princeton University professor has published a book advocating deciding who shall live and who shall die based on their "quality of life."[11]

It is important to note that there is a difference between Western medical ethics and Judaism. Western ethics put great stress on the principle of autonomy; our body is ours to control and thus we can decide what to do with it. Judaism, on the other hand, believes that our role is that of a guardian (*shomer*) of a body that belongs to Hashem. This philosophical difference can lead to different approaches on the part of medical professionals and the family. Involvement of a halachic authority familiar with medical ethics issues can help lead to easier cooperation.[12]

It is clear that actively ending a life is antithetical to the principles of Judaism. Ending the life of a dying person is considered murder.[13] Providing oxygen, food, and water to even a dying person is considered a basic need. Therefore, bringing about death by not providing these items is also considered a form of murder.[14]

Rabbi Moshe Isserles, however, on the basis at least in part on the indirect actions of the maidservant, states in his gloss on the *Shulchan Aruch*[15] that one may do certain indirect actions. One example given in the gloss is that one may stop the banging noise of chopping wood in the vicinity of the *goses* even if it seems that the noise is keeping him alive. While it is hard at times to find the modern-day corollaries of the examples given, this principle is used in individual cases to allow indirect action such as not restarting a ventilator that has stopped.[16, 17]

There is not uniformity of opinion on many of these matters and much will depend on the specifics of the case. Especially in diseases where eventual demise is expected, involvement of a halachic authority in advance can prevent these difficult decisions from being made in a pressured manner.

After the End

The death of a child is experienced as one of the hardest deaths for a family to cope with. Deaths of the generations above us are expected; deaths of the generations below us are not. The death can have an impact on all members of the family.

Parents are generally the ones most affected. Grief tends to make people feel completely disoriented; day runs into night, and days get completely mixed up with each other. The Jewish laws of mourning reflect this process. During the first step, called *onen*,[18] a person is exempt from all positive commandments. This exemption reflects that a person is not able to cope with outside obligations.

The process of sitting *shiva*[19] is designed to allow the family to talk about the deceased. Parents who have lost a child report that this step is *very* important to them. Visitors should allow them to talk as much, or as little, as they want. Even after *shiva* is over, people should not hesitate to mention the child who died. He or she will always remain in the parents' memory.

In practice, the parents may not always be available to the surviving children during the *shiva*. It can be helpful for a relative who is not sitting *shiva*, or a close friend, to take responsibility for the young siblings. Not all laws of mourning apply to young children. Some adult expressions of mourning may be completely inappropriate for a child; others may give the child a sense of participating. It is important to recognize that children will experience intense emotions but express them differently. Therefore, what to ask of children during *shiva* should be discussed with a halachic authority. It can also be helpful to discuss with the child's teacher or school counselor whether a young child should return to school during the *shiva*, and how his or her peers should become involved in the mitzvah of comforting the mourner.

Many terminal genetic conditions involve years of deterioration and severe disability. Caring for the disabled child affects—and potentially limits—the family in many ways. With the child's death, the family must make a rather sudden transition back to a "normal" lifestyle. Doing so can be disorienting. It can also trigger a sense of relief—leading to ambivalence or guilt at "benefiting" from the child's death.

The halachic mourning period for any relative other than a parent continues for 30 days. However, the emotional mourning process continues through life. To help families cope with the death, the following is a list of dos and don'ts.

- Stay in touch with the family. Keep phoning a long time after the loss. Be prepared for the fact that at times the family does not feel like talking. However, the fact that you cared enough to call means a lot. If you are afraid that your call might come at the wrong time, consider email messages or written cards that can be dealt with at their convenience.

- Continue to invite the family to the celebrations that you would have invited them to in the past. While it may seem to you that it will be hurtful for them to be reminded about others who are still alive, not inviting them only increases the isolation that the family feels. On the other hand, don't pressure them to come and don't be insulted if they say no. Each family has to determine their own pace of feeling comfortable with the company of large, happy crowds. Realize that, devastating as it is, the loss of a child does not generally deprive a person of his or her capacity for happiness.

- Offer them opportunities to take part in community activities. However, do not overwhelm them with responsibilities in the hope that it will "get their minds off their loss." Here too the family members have to be the ones to determine the pace.

- Don't forget all the family members. While fathers and mothers may express their emotions differently, they are both mourning. Siblings are also suffering the loss—both the loss of their brother or sister and the loss of their parents' attention as the parents deal with their loss. Children are less likely to express their feelings unless an outlet is offered. If they resist, don't push them, but leave an "open door." Siblings also need to feel normal among their friends—most youngsters don't like to be different. The death of a sibling makes them different.

- Friends may be afraid to approach their bereaved peers. If your child's friend is mourning, speak to your child about how to approach the subject, express sympathy, and offer friendship.

- When the family is ready, help them find an appropriate memorial for their child. While setting up some form of *tzedakah* or *chesed* project is chosen by many families, let them decide what and when without pressure.

- Offer specific help: picking up the other children from school, taking them to after-school or social activities, shopping, or preparing meals for the family. Don't be insulted if the answer is no, and don't hesitate to offer again. These offers tend to come frequently during *shiva*, but the need will continue.

- Don't hesitate to refer to the deceased child by name. Parents like to hear about the child. While talking about them brings up the loss, it also helps keep their memories alive.
- Don't try to give answers as to why this happened. The truth is that no one really knows. The book of *Iyov* (Job) illustrates that this is not the proper way to console people.
- Don't say you understand what they are going through. You don't. Even if you have dealt with your own family tragedy, no two people are the same. Your role is to listen, not to explain.
- Don't try to point out to the family the "positive aspect" of what happened. This is particularly true for children who have had an ongoing decline. It is natural for people on the outside to feel like this is "all for the good" and, in fact, the family may feel some measure of relief at some point. The example in the Torah is Aharon's reaction to the death of his sons. His response was to keep silent.[20] He did not feel that he had to find the positive aspect. The blessing recited upon hearing about death and bad news is that God is the true judge. That is acceptance enough that Hashem has some reason for this to happen, not that we know what it is.

Support Groups (in the hopes that they are never needed)
Donald Alan Harris Healing Hearts Bereavement Program
Chai Lifeline
Internet: www.chailifeline.org
The Bereaved Parents' Network
Care for the Family
Freepost, Cardiff CF15 7GZ222
Phone: 129 2081 0800
Internet: www.careforthefamily.org.uk
Compassionate Friends
Internet: www.compassionatefriends.org
Loss of A Child
Internet: www.lossofachild.org

1. Except for those genetic diseases such as Bloom syndrome or ataxia-telangiectasia where the cause of death is cancer.

2. H. Davies, Living with dying: families coping with a child who has a neurodegenerative genetic disorder. *Axone* 1996; 18:38–44.

3. R. Schnell, Helping parents cope with the dying child with a genetic disorder. *Journal of Clinical Child & Adolescent Psychology* 1974: 3: 34–35.

4. *Shulchan Aruch, Orach Chaim* 329:3–4. See also the Biur Halacha there for further discussion of the importance of even temporary life.

5. Ibid.

6. *Semachot* 1:1–4.

7. *Yoreh Deah* 339:1.

8. *Iggrot Moshe, Yoreh Deah* 2:174:1.

9. A summary of the difference of approach can be found in B. L. Gracer, What the Rabbis heard: deafness in the Mishnah. *Disabilities Studies Quarterly* 2003; 23:192–205.

10. E. Verhagen and P. J. J. Sauer, The Groningen Protocol—Euthanasia in Severely Ill Newborns. *N Engl J Med* 2005; 352:959–62.

11. P. Singer. *Rethinking Life and Death*. New York: St. Martin's Griffin, 1994.

12. Questions can be sent to Machon Schlesinger, www.medethics.org.il.

13. *Shulchan Aruch, Yoreh Deah* 339:1. See also discussion by Rav Eliezer Waldenberg in Tzitz Eliezer 5 Ramat Rachel 29.

14. A. Steinberg, Habasis Hahilchati leHatzaat chok hacholeh hanoteh lamut. *Assia*. Available at www.medethics.org.il.

15. *Yoreh Deah* 339:1.

16. *Techumim*, Vol. II, pp. 304–5. For an opposing view, see Rabbi Eliyah Katz, *Techumim*, Volume III, page 536.

17. *Iggrot Moshe, Choshen Mishpat* 2:73:1.

18. From death until the burial.

19. The seven-day mourning period. This starts from the burial (generally with the part of the day after the burial counting as day one) and ends in the morning of the seventh day.

20. *Vayikra* 10:3.

Concluding Remarks

One of the underlying fears about increasing genetic knowledge is that it will reveal that all is controlled by our genes. This would appear to contradict the notion of free will. It would seem to indicate that "nature," what we inherit, is more important than "nurture," what we are exposed to.

Interestingly, this is not a new debate. The Talmud in *Shabbat* 156a makes the statement that "One who is born under Mars will be 'bloody.'" At the time of the Talmud, astrology was a science. One's fate was thought to be determined by the stars. The overarching statement of the Talmud, however, is followed by a discussion by a number of sages. Rav Ashi explains that being "bloody" can mean that one will become a doctor,[1] a thief, a butcher, or a *mohel*, all professions that have a "bloody" component. This is the aspect that is determined. However, the individual still has the choice of expressing it through positive or negative outlets.

The talmudic passage continues with a debate between Rabbi Chanina and Rabbi Yochanan as to whether, even if astrology has an impact on the rest of the world, perhaps it does not apply to Jews. The debate is followed by a midrashic account of Avraham turning to Hashem to say he has seen, based on astrology, that he will not have a son. Hashem then tells Avraham to ignore the astrology; it does not have an impact on the children of Israel. Rashi points out that prayer and good deeds can change the outcome.

This message that prayer and good deeds can change an outcome is the one with which I wish to "end" this book. No, not every individual case can currently be cured by prayer alone. However, by focusing on the good that can be derived from genetic knowledge, and using the caution that the introspection of prayer should give us, we can help ensure that genetic knowledge is used only for good causes.

It is clear that "end" is a misnomer, since there will continue to be new discoveries all the time. Even in areas where knowledge is well established, this book has touched upon them, not discussed them in complete detail. It is thus fitting to "end" with the statement that finishes many works of Torah:

תם ולא נשלם שבח לקל בורא עולם

315

"Finished but not complete, praise to the Creator of the World." By remembering that there is a Creator, we can retain the humility needed to use genetic knowledge for the good.

---

1. The term *umna* means "bloodletter," which was one form of medical care at the time.

Index of Jewish and Halachic Concepts